AF556497

Nematology

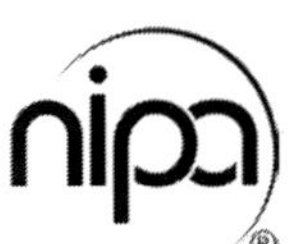

NIPA GENX ELECTRONIC RESOURCES & SOLUTIONS P. LTD.
New Delhi-110 034

Nematology
Fundamentals & Applications

2nd Fully Revised and Enlarged Edition

E.I. JONATHAN, Ph.D., PDF (USA)
(Retd.) Director
Centre for Plant Protection Studies
Tamil Nadu Agricultural University
Coimbatore - 641003, Tamil Nadu, India

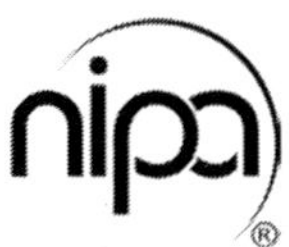

NIPA GENX ELECTRONIC RESOURCES & SOLUTIONS P. LTD.
New Delhi-110 034

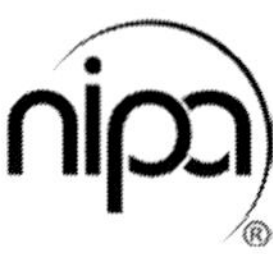

NIPA GENX ELECTRONIC RESOURCES & SOLUTIONS P. LTD.

101,103, Vikas Surya Plaza, CU Block
L.S.C. Market, Pitam Pura, New Delhi-110 034
Ph : +91 11 27341616, 27341717, 27341718
E-mail: newindiapublishingagency@gmail.com
www: www.nipabooks.com

For customer assistance, please contact
Phone: + 91-11-27 34 17 17
Fax: + 91-11-27 34 16 16
E-Mail: feedbacks@nipabooks.com

ISBN: 978-93-91383-37-4

Composed and Designed by NIPA.

Foreword

Nematodes are a primitive group of invertebrates, most diversified and highly developed pseudocoelomate group of animals. Nematodes can live under varied conditions; they are known to occur where ever life can exist: from arctic to tropics and from mountains to oceans. They may be free living in soil or water (fresh, marine and brackish) or may live as parasites on animals, human beings and plants. *Caenorhabditis elegans*, a free living transparent nematode in temperate soils is the model organism for studies on developmental biology, worldwide. *C. elegans* is the first multicellular organism to have its genome completely sequenced.

Plant parasitic nematodes are a complex, diverse group of micro round worms that occur in all environments. Plant parasitic nematodes are recognized as serious pests on crop plants in recent years. Comprehensive research effort on plant parasitic nematodes was initiated in late 1950's in our country. Reports on the molya disease of wheat and barley in Rajasthan in 1958, occurrence of potato cyst nematode in 1961 in the Nilgiri hills and endemics of root-knot nematode damage in wide variety of crops underscore the seriousness of nematode pests. The damage caused by nematodes is often overlooked and confused with nutritional disorders, since the symptoms are not explicit unlike that of insect pests and pathogens.

Realizing the importance of nematodes as limiting factors in agricultural production, Agricultural Nematology was included in the curriculum at the undergraduate level in many Agricultural Universities. A separate department for Plant Nematology was started in Tamil Nadu Agricultural University, Coimbatore during the year 1981 with the objectives to pursue research, education and extension activities related to Nematology. Nematology is also widely covered in revised syllabus of Zoology by UGC governed colleges.

There is a paucity of text books in Nematology for undergraduate students. This book entitled "Nematology Fundamentals and Applications" is designed as a text book, to give a comprehensive account of all essential aspects of Nematology. This book will surely serve as an eye opener for students of Nematology, Zoology and Molecular biology. It will enable them to understand the biology of nematodes besides generating interest among young scientists. Elaborate coverage on nematode pests of important crop plants should serve as a helpful reference to all agricultural technicians and extension functionaries to identify and suggest appropriate recommendation for the management of the nematodes in the field level.

I am confident that this book will serve as a vade-mecum for Nematologists, Botanists, Zoologists and Plant Protection workers. I appreciate the efforts taken by Dr. E. I. Jonathan, Director, Centre for Plant Protection Studies, TNAU, Coimbatore to compile this book.

-sd-

(P. Murugesa Boopathi)

Vice Chancellor

Preface

Nematodes are a complex, diverse group of round worms that occur worldwide in essentially all the environments. Plant parasitic nematodes are recognized as serious pests of crop plants in recent years. The world-wide annual crop loss due to these obligate parasites have been estimated as $ 78 billion. The damage caused by nematodes are often overlooked. They are hidden enemies and the associated symptoms can also be attributed to nutritional and water related disorders. The epidemics of sugarbeet sickness due to cyst nematode, yellow disease of black pepper, molya disease on wheat and barley, the ear-cockle disease on wheat and others have led to the recognition of the science Plant Nematology as an important branch of Agricultural Sciences. The recognition of nematodes as serious detevrrents to crop productivity was felt in India only in the 1961, when Dr. Jones from Germany reported the menace of potato cyst problems were identified in important crop plants. Compared to other disciplines of crop protection, Plant Nematology is the youngest deserving tremendous support to strengthen the discipline.

The Department of Nematology at Tamil Nadu Agricultural University, Coimbatore has been in the forefront and has provided leadership in strengthening the discipline of Nematology in the country. Recently, Nematology has been included in the curriculum of few Agricultural Universities in India and as such, there is a paucity of text book in Nematology to cater the needs of students. In this direction, a sincere attempt has been made to bring out a comprehensive text book dealing with the relevant aspects of the subject, Agricultural Nematology.

This book has been written as a text book primarily keeping in view of the requirements of undergraduate students of agriculture, horticulture and post-graduates specializing on Nematology and Entomology dealing with plant parasitic nematodes. This book provides a brief account of historical background including the developments in India and abroad, details of morphology, anatomy and taxonomy of plant parasitic nematodes, relevant nematological techniques and focus on nematode problems in important agricultural and horticultural crop and their management.

The book also provides a brief account of Caenorhabditis elegans which is being used as a biological model in most of the biological research. The book will also be useful to those who are preparing for competitive examinations conducted by various central and state government agencies for recruitment. Every attempt has been made to provide necessary information from the view point of students dealing biological sciences.

The help rendered by Miss. S.Santhi, Assistant Professor, Agricultural Entomology and N.Nivetha, Assistant Professor, Agricultural Entomology, The Indian Agriculture College, Radhapuram in assisting the proof correction is gratefully acknowledged.

Place: Tamil Nadu (Author)

Date: 31.07.2022

Contents

Glossary

A

A : A ratio calculated by dividing the length of the nematode by its maximum width.

Abduce : To head away or way to

Abduct : Non living

Acanthiform : Look like thorn shape

Acetylcholine : Chemical transmitter of nerve and nerve-muscle impulses in animals.

Acute : Sharp pointed

Active ingredient(a.i) : Chemicals in a product that are responsible for the pesticidal effect.

Adanal bursa : Bursa enclose a part of the tail

Aerolated : The transverse line present in the lateral fields

Aestivation : Dormant during unfavourable dry condition

Alae : Longitudinal thickening of cuticle forming wing like expansion (longitudinal alae, cervical alae, caudal alae and bursa)

Alate : Possessing lateral field.

Ambifenestrate : The occurrence of two openings in the vulval cone which are seperated by the vulval bridge as observed in some species of *Heterodera.*

Amphid : Paired sensory organ located at the anterior.

Amphidelphic : Female with two ovaries one situated anterior and other posterior to the vulva.

Annulation : A transverse depression, appearing as a line on the cuticle.

Annules : Ring like markings.

Anus : The posterior opening of the digestive tract.

Antagonistic plant : Plants having antagonistic effect on the nematodes. They are also known as enemy plants. Marigold and Pangola grass are examples for such plants.

Antidode : A practical treatment including first aid used in the treatment of pesticide poisoning or some other poison in the body.

Aquatic : Organism living in a water habitat.

Arc : A bow like curvature (Arcuate).

Atrophy : Arrested development.

Atropine : An antidote used to treat organophosphate and carbamate poisoning.

Attenuate : Slender, thin, elongate.

Axis : A straight line passing through the body.

B

B : A ratio calculated by dividing the total body length by the length of the oesophagus measured from the anterior end of the body.

Basement membrane : A layer which separates the innermost layer of the cuticle from the hypodermis.

Basal bulb : Posterior portion of oesophagus which may be a distinct bulb like structure or a lobe overlapping the intestine.

Biotype : A subdivision of a race.

Bisexual : Distinct, separate male and female individuals.

Bilaterally symmetry : This condition is referred to those organisms where the body can be divided into two equal halves by passing a dorso-ventral plane through the body axis.

Blind bud : An abortive flower bud due to nematode infestation.

Bloat : The disease caused by *Ditylenchus dipsaci* on onion and also known as onion bloat.

Body cavity : Hollow tube containing internal organs.

Buccal cavity : It is also referred as stoma. It connects oral opening with anterior portion of the oesophagus.

Bursa : Wing like lateral expansion on the cuticle in the male tail

Bullae : Knob like structure located within the vulval cone of cysts of *Herterodera* near the underbridge or fenestra.

C

C : A ratio calculated by dividing the total length by length of the tail.

Cardia : Oesophageal intestinal valve.

Caudal glands : Three or five glands located in the tail region of the nematode.

Caudal alae : Bursa.

Cephalic framework : A subcuticular framework that supports the lip region and to which the stylet and associated muscles are attached.

Choline esterase : An enzyme of the animal body neccessary for proper nerve function that is inhibited or damaged by organo-phosphate and carbamate pesticides.

Circumoesophageal : It is also known as nerve ring. This nerve ring **commissure** encircles the oesophagus as a band of nerve fibres. It is associated with the central nervous system of the nematode having nerve connections both from anterior and posterior part of the nematode.

Circomyarian : Round muscle cells and the muscle fibres in the cells surrounding the cytoplasm.

Coelomyarian : 'U' shaped cells in which muscle fibre are adjacent and perpendicular to the hypodermis and extend along the sides of the muscle cell of varying distances.

Cloaca : In male a common opening empties the digestive and reproductive system.

Crescent : Sickle shaped.

Cortex : The outermost layer of the cuticle.

Cuticle : The non-cellular external layer of a nematode produced by the hypodermis. Cuticle covers the nematode body.

Cyst : Matured female body become thick and resistant as seen in the genus *Heterodera* and *Globodera.*

D

Didelphic : Two ovaries.

Diorchic : Two testis.

E

Egg mass : Eggs laid in gelatinous matrix.

Emulsifiable : Concentrated pesticide formulation containing **concentrate** organic solvent and emulsifier to facilitate emulsification with water.

Excretory pore : Opening through which the waste products of excretory system emptied.

F

Fenestra : A window like opening found in the vulval cone of *Heterodera.*

Filariasis : A disease caused by the filarial worm *Wuchereria bancrofti* in human beings and the disease is also known as elephantiasis.

Foliar nematode : The nematode which feeds on the aerial parts.

Free living nematodes : Non parasitic nematodes devoid of stylet.

Fumigation : Application of toxic gas to an area to control various pests. For nematode control frequently applied as a liquid using soil injector.

G

Gall : Swelling.

Gastrula : An early embryo composed of a hollow two-layered cup-shaped structure derived from the blastula.

Genital Papillae : Tactile or sensory organs located on the tail.

Giant cell : Also known as syncytium. At the feeding site of the nematode 6 - 8 multinucleate abnormal big cells are formed due to the infestation of root-knot and cyst nematodes. These giant cells have thick cytoplasm and provide nourishment to the developing larvae.

Gravid female : An adult female containing eggs.

Gubernaculum : Sclerotized piece of plate found in male nematodes which guides and deflects the spicules.

Guiding ring : A cuticularized structure which surrounds and guides the stylet as found in *Xiphinema* and *Longidorus*.

H

Hatching factor : External factor which stimulates the hatching of eggs.

Hemizonid : Refractive, biconvex, semicircular lens-like structure situated between the cuticle and the hypodermis on the ventral side of the body just anterior to the excretory pore and believed to be associated with the nervous system.

Hypertrophy : Abnormal increase in cell size.

Hyperplasia : Abnormal increase in cell number.

I

Incisures : Longitudinal cuticular clefts which divide the lateral fields.

Infective juvenile : The larval stage of the nematode that can penetrate the host.

Inter sex : An individual which exhibits both male and female characters.

Isthmus : Narrow portion of the oesophagus found between the median bulb and the basal bulb.

J

Juvenile : The larval stage of nematode or immature stage.

L

L : The overall length of a nematode in millimeters.

Labial : Pertaining to or located on the lips.

Labial disc : A raised area in the cuticle of the most anterior annule of some species of *Criconemoides*.

Lateral field : A pair of laterally located longitudinal cuticular markings located above the lateral hypodermal chords.

Lumen : Triradiate canal of the duct of the oesophagus.

M

Mesentron : The intestine.

Metacorpus : Also known as median bulb. A broad muscular portion of the oesophagus located in the middle portion of the oesophagus.

Microvilli : Finger like projections of the plasma membrane which increases the surface area of the intenstine for effective absorption.

Migratory : A parasitic nematode which feeds on the **ectoparasite** host from outside while remaining in the rhizosphere e.g. *Tylenchorhynchus.*

Migratory : A parasitic nematode which enters a host, **endoparasite** feeds internally, move freely inside the tissue e.g. *Radopholus similis* on banana and *Hirschmanniella oryzae* on rice.

Monodelphic : Single ovary as found in *Pratylenchus*.

Monorchic : Single testis.

Mucron : Small projection or point in nematode tail.

N

NEPO : Nematode transmitted virus with polyhedral particles.

NETU : Nematode transmitted virus with tubular particles.

Nematode wool : A mass of desiccated *Ditylenchus* found in some plant tissues.

Nurse cell : Transformed cell due to nematode host interaction in the case of citrus nematode infestation which has thick cell wall and enlarged nucleus.

O

Odontostylet : Originates in the oesophagus wall. Also known as onchiostylet.

Opisthodelphic : Having a single ovary situated posterior to the vulva.

Oocyte : An immature female gamete.

P

Papillae : Sensory structures located in the lip region, 16 in number known as cephalic papillae tactile in function and also act as chemoreceptor.

Phasmid : A pair of pore-like sensory structures located in the posterior region of the nematode which comes under the class Secernentea. Main functions are chemoreception, mechano- reception and thermoreception.

Platymyarian : A flat type of muscle cell with contractile elements limited to the base lying close to the epidermis.

Posterior cuticular : Also known as perineal pattern. Finger print like pattern formed due to the cuticular striations or markings in the perineum region of the adult female of *Meloidogyne.*

Preadult : The fourth stage juvenile just before the adult stage.

Predatory nematode : The nematode which feeds on the plant parasitic nematode like the genus *Mononchus*.

Procorpus : The anterior narrow tube like portion of the oesophagus located between the base of the stoma and the metacorpus.

R

Rachis : An axial or column.

Rectal glands : Glands located in the rectal region. In the genus *Meloidogyne* these rectal glands secretes gelatinous mucopolysaccharide in which eggs are deposited as a mass.

Renette : A ventral cell present in the excretory system of some nematodes.

Rhizosphere : The area of soil surrounding plant roots.

S

S : Stylet length/body diameter measured at the base of stylet.

Scutellum : Enlarged phasmid found in some species of the family Hoplolaimidae.

Sedentary : The nematode capable of entering the **endoparasite** host as juvenile, migrate to fix a feeding site and become immobile eg. root-knot and cyst nematodes.

Semifenestrae : A pair of openings in the vulval cone of the cysts in the genus *Heterodera* which is separated by the vulval bridge.

Seminal vesicle : A portion of the male reproductive tract which functions as a temporary storage of sperm.

Setae : Enlarged cuticular structures mostly located around the oral opening and they are tactile in function.

Sexual dimorphism : Morphological differences between the male and female.

Sheath : A covering of a structure as found in some species of nematodes where the moulted cuticle remain without shedding and covers the nematode body.

Spermatheca : An enlarged portion of the female gonad found between the oviduct and uterus which stores the sperms.

Spermatocyte : A cell giving rise to sperm cells or spermatozoa.

Spicule : A pair of sclerotised male copulatory organ.

Stomatostylet : A stylet evolved by the fusion of the walls of the stoma as commonly found in the members of the order Tylenchida.

Stomodeum : The anterior portion of the digestive system formed by the invagination of the cuticle.

Stylet : Also known as spear. Scleortised needle like feeding structure located in the buccal cavity of the nematodes. Stylet helps to penetrate the host and to feed on them.

T

Tail : The posterior portion of the nematode from the anal opening to the tail tip.

Telamon : Rigid sclerotised portion of the cloacal wall which apparently guides the spicules from the spicular pouch into the cloaca. eg. Stronglylids.

Testis : Male reproductive organ.

Trap crop : A crop in which the nematode can penetrate but they cannot reach the maturity stage.

Triploblastic : Possessing three layers as ectoderm, mesoderm and endoderm.

U

Underbringe : A structure extending across the vulval cone of *Heterodera* cysts below and parallel to the vulval bridge.

V

V : The location of the vulval opening in the body length of the nematode and expressed in percentage.

Vas deferens : The portion of the male reproductive system leading from the vas efferentia to the seminal vesicle and ejaculatory duct.

Vector : An agent which transmit the virus disease. *Xiphenema index* transmit fan leaf virus disease in grapevine plants.

Vulva : The external opening of the female reproductive system and its position in nematodes are important taxonomic character.

Vulval bridge : A narrow connection across the fenestra of vulva cones in the cyst of some species of the genus *Heterodera* which form two semifenestrae.

Vulval cone : The elevated portion of the posterior portion of the *Heterodera* cysts.

1

Introduction

Agricultural crops are being affected by a wide range of organisms such as insects, mites, fungi, bacteria etc. Another important and unseen enemy is known as plant parasitic nematodes. The study on nematodes is known as Nematology.

Nematology is an important branch of biological science, which deals with a complex, diverse group of round worms known as **Nematodes** that occur worldwide in essentially all environments. Nematodes are also known as eelworms in Europe, nemas in the United States and round worms by zoologists. Many species are important parasites of plants and animals, whereas others are beneficial to agriculture and the environment. Nematodes that are parasites of man and animals are called helminths and the study is known as Helminthology. The name nematode was derived from Greek words nema (thread) and oides (resembling). This book focuses primarily on plant parasitic nematodes, their morphology, anatomy, nematological techniques, taxonomy, classification based on their feeding habits, symptom of damage to crops, interaction with other microorganisms, biology of important nematodes *viz., Meloidogyne, Heterodera, Rotylenchulus, Tylenchulus* and *Radopholus* and nematode pests of important crops and their management.

Annual crop losses due to these obligate parasites have been estimated to be about $78 billion worldwide and $8 billion for U.S. growers. The estimated annual crop loss in Tamil Nadu is around Rs. 200 crores.

The soil in a hectare of agroecosystem typically contains billions of plant parasitic as well as beneficial nematodes. The damage to plants caused by nematodes is often overlooked because the associated symptoms, including slow growth, stunting and yellowing can also be attributed to nutritional and water related disorders.

Importance of Nematodes in Agriculture

In the United States, the nematodes are known to cause six per cent loss in field crops ($100 million /year), 12 per cent loss in fruits and nuts ($225 million/

year), 11 per cent loss in vegetables ($267 million/year) and 10 per cent loss in ornamentals ($60 million/year).

In India, the cereal cyst nematode, *Heterodera avenae* causes the **'molya'** disease of wheat and barley in Rajasthan, Punjab, Haryana, Himachal pradesh and Jammu and Kashmir. The loss due to this nematode is about 32 million rupees in wheat and 25 million rupees for barley in Rajasthan State alone.

The seed gall nematode, *Anguina tritici* causes the **'ear-cockle'** disease of wheat in North India. This nematode along with the bacterium, *Clavibacter tritici* causes **'tundu'** or **'yellow slime'** disease. The overall damage is about one per cent, but in severe infestation, the loss may even go up to 80 per cent. The annual loss due to this nematode in North India is about 10,000 tonnes of wheat costing 70 million rupees.

The potato cyst nematodes, *Globodera rostochiensis* and *G. pallida* are serious problem in the Nilgiris and Kodaikanal Hills in potato. About 3,000 hectares are infested by this nematode. Total failure of the crop has been recorded under severe infestation.

The root-lesion nematode, *Pratylenchus coffeae* is a serious pest of coffee in South India. About 1,000 hectares are infested by this nematode. Annual loss is about 20 million rupees.

The burrowing nematode, *Radopholus citrophilus* causes **'spreading decline'** of citrus in Florida. *R. similis* causes **'pepper yellows'** in Indonesia and **'banana rhizome rot'** in various parts of the world. This nematode is a serious pest in banana, coconut, arecanut and ginger. It is also responsible for **'slow wilt'** of pepper in Karnataka.

The citrus nematode, *Tylenchulus semipenetrans* is responsible for **'slow decline'** disease of citrus. It is suggested that the citrus nematode is also one among the factors responsible for **'die-back disease'** of citrus trees in India. The total annual reduction in the citrus crop due to the nematode infestation is estimated at 15 per cent. In severe infestation, the life span of citrus trees are very much reduced. The nematode infestation symptoms are clearly seen in trees with the age group of 5-10 years. The severe infestation in acid lime gardens are observed in Perambalur district of Tamil Nadu.

The reniform nematode, *Rotylenchulus reniformis* has been reported to cause 14.9, 8.1, 6.0, 13.2, and 8.7 per cent loss in yield of cotton, maize, finger millet, cowpea and black gram respectively.

The root-knot nematodes, *Meloidogyne* spp. produce galls on roots of many vegetable crops, pulses, some fruit crops, tobacco and ornamental crops and lead to severe yield loss. This nematode is mostly polyphagous and attack more that 3000 species of plants.

The avoidable yield losses due to *M.incognita* is as follows

Crop	% loss
Bhendi	28.0
Brinjal	33.0
Tomato	35.0
French bean	43.0
Cowpea	28.0
Peas	20.0

In severe infestation, 60-80 per cent loss in yield was observed in the crops.

Estimated annual losses due to nematodes for selected world crops

Crops	Number of estimates per crop	Food and Agriculture Organization production estimates (1000 MT)	Estimated yield losses due to Nematodes (%)
Banana	78	2 097	19.7
Barley	49	171 635	6.3
Cassava	25	129 020	8.4
Citrus	102	56 100	14.2
Cocoa	13	1 660	10.5
Coffee	36	5 210	15.0
Corn	125	449 255	10.2
Cotton (lint)	85	17 794	10.7
Field bean	70	19 508	10.9
Oat	37	43 355	4.2
Peanut	69	20 611	12.0
Potato	141	312 209	12.2
Rice	64	469 959	10.0
Sorghum	53	71 698	6.9
Soybean	91	89 893	10.6
Sugarbeet	51	293 478	10.9
Sugarcane	65	935 769	15.3
Sweet potato	67	117 337	10.2
Tea	16	2 218	8.2
Tobacco	92	6 205	14.7
Wheat	89	521 682	7.0

The examples are only a small portion of nematode problem in India. Besides this direct damage, they also associate with bacteria, fungi and viruses to cause complex diseases.

2

History of Plant Nematology

In light of the high population of nematodes, N.A. Cobb (1915) who is considered to be the father of American Nematology, provided a dramatic description of the abundance of nematodes. He stated, "if all the matter in the universe except the nematodes were swept away, our world still would be dimly recognisable. We would find its mountain tops, valleys, rivers, lakes and oceans represented by a film of nematodes." The Papyrus Ebers suggested a knowledge of the human intestinal parasite, *Ascaris lumbricoides* and the tissue parasite, *Dracunculus medinensis*. In early Egyptian writings also these two human parasites have been described. In 1956, Borellus recorded his observations "Vinegar eels" the microbivorous or free living nematode occurring in most vinegar at that time. The statement "sowed cockle, reaped no corn" in Shakespeare's "Love's Labour's Lost", act 4, scene 3, as suggested by Thorne (1961) possibly the first record of plant parasitic nematodes in 1549. The nematode that Thorne suspected to be in that reference actually was described by Needham in 1743. Subsequently, discovery of microscope and developments in various disciplines of science led to the discovery of plant parasitic nematodes and the disease caused by them. Some of the important milestones on the history of plant nematology are listed below in chronological order.

1743- Needham - Discovery of wheat seed gall nematode, *Anguina tritici,* the first plant parasitic nematode to come to the attention of the early investigators.

1855- Berkeley - Determination of root-knot nematode, *Meloidogyne* spp. to cause root galls on cucumber plants in greenhouse in England.

1857- Kuhn - Reported the stem and bulb nematode, *Ditylenchus dipsaci* infesting the heads of teassel.

1859- Schacht - Reported the sugarbeet cyst nematode, *Heterodera schachtii* from Germany.

1873- Butschli - Descriptions of the morphology of free-living nematodes.

1884- de Man - Taxonomic monograph of soil and fresh water nematodes of the Netherlands.

1889- Atkinson and Neal - Publication about the root-knot nematodes in the United States.

1892- Atkinson - First report of root-knot nematode and *Fusarium* complex in vascular wilt of cotton.

1907- N.A. Cobb - Joined the USDA and considered to be the Father of American Nematology.

1914- N.A. Cobb - Contributions to the Science of Nematology.

1918- N.A. Cobb - Development of methods and apparatus used in Nematology.

1933- T. Goodey - Book on "Plant parasitic nematodes and the disease they cause".

1934- Filipjev - Book on "Nematodes that are important for Agriculture" translated from Russian to English in 1941 by S. Stekhovan under the title "A Manual of Agricultural Helminthology".

1943- Carter - Description of nematicidal value of D-D which is used in the era of soil fumigation.

1945- Christie - Description of the nematicidal value of EDB.

1948- Allen - Taught the World's first formal university course in Nematology at the University of California, Berkeley.

1950- Oostenbrink - Wrote a Book on "The Potato Nematode, A dangerous parasite to Potato Monoculture."

1951- Christie and Perry - Role of ectoparasites as plant pathogens. T. Goodey - Wrote a book on "Soil and fresh water nematodes". Food and Agriculture Organisation of the United Nations organised the first International Nematology course and Symposium held at Rothamsted Experiment Station, England.

1955- European Society of Nematologists founded.

1956- Nematologica - The first journal published exclusively for Nematology from The Netherlands.

1961- Society of Nematologists founded in the United States.

1967- Organization of Tropical American Nematologists founded.

1969- Journal of Nematology was first published by the Society of Nematologists, USA.

1973- Nematologica Mediterranea - published from Italy.

1978- Revue de Nematologie published from France.

1930s - 1990s - Barron, Duddingeon, Mankau, Linford, Sayre and Zuckerman- provided an insight on the Biological control of plant-parasitic nematodes. Enhanced understanding of antagonists and related biology enhancing the potential for practical biocontrol.

1940s - 1990s-Van Gundy-Advancement in survival mechanisms of nematodes which provided fundamental knowledge and facilitated practical control.

1950s - 1990s-Triantaphyllou-Provided advancement in Cyto-genetics, mode of reproduction / sexuality - and information data base for genetics / molecular research. Enhanced understanding of evolution and taxa interrelationships.

1950s - 1990s - Caveness, Jones, Oostenbrink, Sasser and Seinhorst -International programme such as International *Meloidogyne* Project - They expanded educational base of nematologists worldwide and provided ecological - taxonomic data base.

1960s - 1990s - Nickle, Poinar and Steiner-Biological control of insects with nematodes.

1960s - 1990s - Brenner, Dougherty and Nicholas-*Caenorhabditis elegans* developmental biology and genetics - model system - provided fundamental information on cell lineage, behaviour, gene function, ageing and overall genome for this model biological system.

In addition to the above, now the research advancement are in progress in the following areas in USA from the year 1990.

- Molecular markers for resistance genes, which provide efficiency of breeding for resistance.
- Molecular analysis of host-parasitic interactions which provides fundamental knowledge on mechanisms of pathogenesis.
- Cloning of resistance genes - Elucidation of the molecular mechanism of resistance
- Transgenic host resistance to plant parasitic nematodes.

History of Nematology in India

Nematology as a separate branch of Agriculture Science in India has been recognised only about 37 years back. The history and development of Nematology in India have been listed below in chronological order.

1901 - Barber first reported root-knot nematode on tea in Devala Estate, Tamil Nadu, South India.

1906 - Butler reported root-knot nematode on black pepper in Kerala.

1913 - Butler reported Ufra disease on rice in Bengal due to

1919 the infestation of *Ditylenchus angustus.*

1926 - Ayyar reported root-knot nematode infestation on

1933 vegetables and other crops in India.

1934 - Dastur reported white tip disease of rice caused by

1936 *Aphelenchoides besseyi* in Central India.

1959 - Prasad, Mathur and Sehgal -reported cereal cyst nematode for the first time from India.

1961 - Nematology laboratory established at Agricultural College and Research Institute, Coimbatore, with the assistance of Rockefeller Foundation and Indian Council of Agricultural Research.

1961 - Jones reported the potato cyst nematode for the first time from Uthagamandalam, Tamil Nadu.

1961 - Nematology unit established at the Central Potato Research Institute, Simla.

1963 - Laboratory for potato cyst nematode research established at Uthagamandalam with the assistance of Indian Council of Agricultural Research.

1964 - First International Nematology Course held at I.A.R.I., New Delhi.

1966 - Nair, Dass and Menon reported the burrowing nematode on banana for the first time from Kerala.

1966 - Division of Nematology established at I.A.R.I., New Delhi.

1968 - First South-East Asian Post-Graduate Nematology course held in India.

1969 - Nematological Society of India founded and first All India Nematology Symposium held at I.A.R.I., New Delhi.

1969- Third South-East Asian Nematology course conducted
1970 at New Delhi.

1971 - Indian Journal of Nematology published.

1971 - Fourth South-East Asian Nematology course at New Delhi.

1972- First All India Nematology Workshop held at I.A.R.I., New Delhi.

1973 - Fifth South-East Asian Nematology course at New Delhi.

1975- Sixth South-East Asian Nematology course at New Delhi.

1976- Summer Institute in Phytonematology held at Allahabad.

1977- Department of Nematology established at Haryana Agricultural University, Hisar.

1977- All India Co-ordinated Research Project (AICRP) on nematode pests of crops and their control started functioning in 14 centres in India with its Project Co-ordinator at I.A.R.I., New Delhi.

1979- M.Sc. (Ag) Plant Nematology course started at Tamil Nadu Agricultural University, Coimbatore.

1979- All India Nematology Workshop and Symposium held at Orissa University of Agriculture and Technology, Bhubaneshwar.

1979- Seventh South-East Asian Nematology course at New Delhi.

1981 - Department of Nematology established at Tamil Nadu Agricultural University, Coimbatore.

1982- Department of Nematology established at Rajendra Agricultural University, Pusa, Bihar.

1983- All India Nematology Workshop and Symposium held at Solan, Himachal Pradesh.

1985- All India Nematology Workshop Symposium held at Udaipur, Rajasthan.

1986- National Conference on Nematology held at I.A.R.I., New Delhi.

1987- All India Nematology Workshop at Govt. Agriculture College Pune.

1987- Group Discussions on Nematological problems of Plantation crops held at Sugarcane Breeding Institute, Coimbatore.

1992- Silver Jubilee Celebration of Division of Nematology, I.A.R.I. New Delhi.

1992- Summer Institute on "Management of Plant Parasitic nematodes in different crops" organised by ICAR at Haryana Agricultural University, Hisar.

1995 - All India Nematology Workshop and National symposium on Nematode problems of India held at I.A.R.I., New Delhi.

1997 - Summer School on "Problems and Progress in Nematology during the past one decade" was organised by ICAR at I.A.R.I., New Delhi.

1998 - Afro-Asian Nematology Conference held during April 1998 at Coimbatore.

1999 - National seminar on "Nematological Research in India : Challenges and preparedness for the new millennium" at C.S. Azad University of Agriculture and Technology, Kanpur.

2000 - National Nematology Symposium on "Integrated Nematode Management" held at OUAT, Bhubaneshwar, Orissa.

2001 - National Congress on "Centenary of Nematology in India: Appraisal and Future plans" at I.A.R.I., New Delhi.

2002 - "Centenary of Nematology in Tamil Nadu" Celebrated at Department of Nematology, Tamil Nadu Agricultural University, Coimbatore.

2003 - Winter School on "Biological control of plant parasitic nematodes" from 2nd to 22nd December, 2003 at Department of Nematology, Tamil Nadu Agricultural University, Coimbatore.

2004 - ICAR sponsored Summer School on 'Recent technologies in the Management of Phytoparasitic nematodes for sustainable agriculture - Sep 8-28, 2004 at CCS, Haryana Agricultural University.

- National Symposium on Paradigms in Nematological Research for biodynamic farming held at Bangalore from November, 17-19, 2004.

2005 - National Symposium on Recent advances and Research priorities in Indian Nematology held at IARI, New Delhi from December, 9-10, 2005.

2006 - Summer school on "Nematode biodiversity, indentification, community dynamics and role of beneficial nematodes in soil health for major cropping systems in relevance to integrated pest management" was held at Division of Nematology, IARI, New Delhi from 7-27 September, 2006.

2007 - Workshop on Nematology in India : Achievements and Opportunities was hled at Division of Nematology, IARI, New Delhi during 5-7th March, 2007.

2007 - National Symposium on Nematology in 21st Century : Emerging Paradigms was helf at Assam Agriculture University, Assam during 22-23 November, 2007.

2010 - National Conference on Innnovtion sin nematoloical research for agricultural sustainability – Chllenges and a roadma ahead, Tamil Nadu Agricultural University, Coimbatore.

2011 - Nematodes: A challenge Under Changing Climate and Agricultural Practices KJJM Animation Centre, Kovalam, Thiruvananthapuram, Kerala, 16-18 November, 2011.

2013 - Nationl Symposium on Nematodes – A Friend and Foe of Agri – Horticultural Crops.Y.S . Parmar University of Horticulture Forestry, Solan, Himachal Pradesh, 31-23 November, 2013.

2015 - Nematode management: A challenge to Indian Agriculture in the changing climate, Yashwantrao Chavan Academy of Development Administration, Pune, 8-10 January, 2015.

2017 - Climate Smart Agriculture for Nematode Management, ICAR-Central Coastal Agricultural Research Institute, Goa, 11-13 January, 2017.

2019 - Nematodes: A threat to food security and farmer's livelihood, Manipur University, Imphal, 11-13 December, 2019.

2021 - The Facets of Innovation and Development of Plant Nematology (Online), Nematological Society of India, IARI, New Delhi (Virtual), 29-30 October, 2021

Reasons for the slow progress of Nematology

1. The nematodes are mostly soil borne organisms which are microscopic and cannot be seen with naked eye.
2. The symptoms of damage caused by nematodes are not specific unlike the damages by insects and other pathogens. The symptoms more or less resemble nutritional disorders.
3. Very recently, the science of Nematology has been included in the curriculum of Agricultural Universities.

4. The extension workers are not trained to identify the nematode problems.
5. Very few nematicides are available in the market and they are costly.
6. The Nematologists available in the country are very few.
7. In many of the Agricultural and Horticultural Colleges nematology research is not carriedout due to non-availability of Namatology.

3

Morphology and Anatomy of Nematodes

Eventhough nematodes occupy nearly every habitat on earth, they are remarkably similar in morphology and life stages. Despite their structural complexity, certain basic principles are common to all nematodes. Nematodes are triploblastic, bilaterally symmetrical, unsegmented, pseudocoelomate, vermiform and colourless animals. The plant parasitic nematodes are slender, elongate, spindle shaped or fusiform, tapering towards both ends and circular in cross section. The length of the nematodes may very from 0.2 mm (*Paratylenchus*) to about 11.0 mm (*Paralongidorus maximus*). Their body width vary from 0.01 to 0.05 mm. In few genera, the females on maturity assume pear shape (*Meloidogyne*), globular shape (*Globodera*), reniform (*Rotylenchulus reniformis*) or saccate (*Tylenchulus semipenetrans*). The swelling increases the reproductive potential of the organism. Radially symmetric traits (triradiate, tetraradiate and hexaradiate) exist in the anterior region. The regions of intestine, excretory and reproductive systems show tendencies towards asymmetry. The nematodes have one or two tubular gonads which open separately in the female and into the rectum in the male which also have the copulatory spicules.

The free living saprophytic nematodes are generally larger in size. The animal and human parasitic helminths may have length of few centimetres to even a meter or more. The helminth parasitising whale fish is about 27 feet long. The study on these animals and human parasites are known as Helminthology.

The following are some examples of Helminths.

1. Filarial worm - *Wuchereria bancrofti*
2. Guinea worm - *Dracunculus medinensis*
3. Round worm - *Ascaris lumbricoides*
4. Tape worm - *Taenia solium*

The nematode body is not divided into definite parts, but certain sub-divisions are given for convenience. The anterior end starts with the head which consists of mouth and pharynx bearing the cephalic papillae or setae. The portion between the head and the base of the oesophagus is known as the neck. Beginning at the anus and extending to the posterior terminus is the tail. Body morphology of a typical plant parasitic nematode is furnished in Fig.1

Longitudinally the body is divided into four regions as dorsal, right lateral, left lateral and ventral. All the natural openings like excretory pore, vulva and anus are located in the ventral region. The nematode body is made up of several distinct body systems. They are the body wall, nervous system, secretory-excretory system, digestive system and reproductive system. Nematodes do not possess a specialised circulatory or respiratory system. The exchange of gases is thought to occur through the cuticle and circulation proceeds through the movement of fluids within the pseudocoelom and by simple diffusion across membranes.

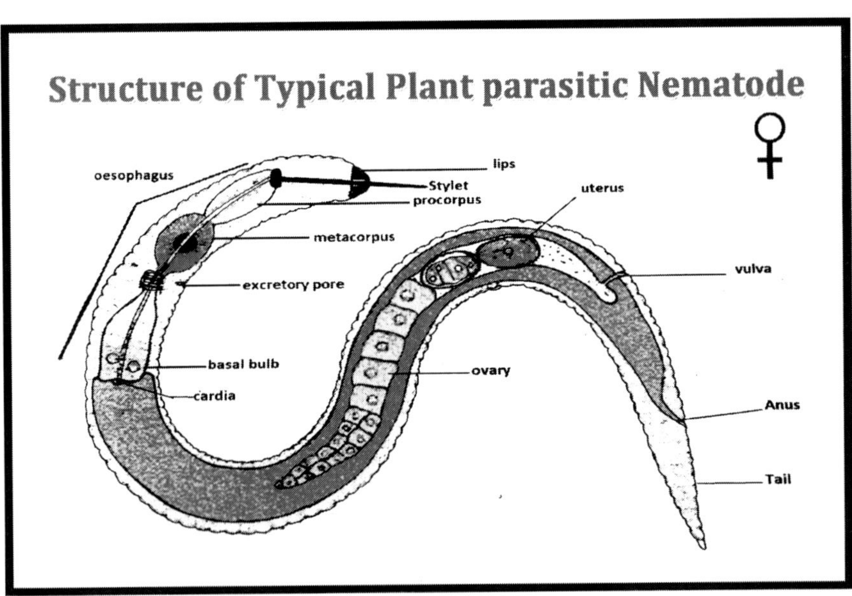

Fig. 1: Morphology of a typical plant parasitic nematode

The following are the characteristics of members of the phylum Nemata

1. Inhabit marine, fresh water and terrestrial environments as free-livers and parasites.
2. Bilaterally symmetrical, triploblastic, unsegmented and pseudo-coelomates.

3. Vermiform, round in cross-section, covered with a three-layered cuticle.
4. Growth accompanied by moulting of juvenile stages, usually four juvenile stages.
5. Oral opening surrounded by 6 lips and 16 sensory structures.
6. Possess unique cephalic sense organs called amphids.
7. Body wall contains only longitudinal muscles connected to longitudinal nerve chords by processes extending from each muscle.
8. Unique excretory system containing gland cells or a set of collecting tubes.
9. Longitudinal nerve chords housed within the thickening of the hypodermis.

Genera of the most common plant parasitic nematodes

1.	Awl nematode	*Dolichodorus* spp.
2.	Cyst nematodes	*Globodera* spp., *Heterodera* spp.
3.	Dagger nematode	*Xiphinema* spp.
4.	White tip nematode	*Aphelenchoides* spp.
5.	Lance nematode	*Hoplolaimus* spp.
6.	Lesion/meadow nematode	*Pratylenchus* spp.
7.	Needle nematode	*Longidorus* spp.
8.	Pin nematode	*Paratylenchus* spp.
9.	Reniform nematode	*Rotylenchulus* spp.
10.	Ring nematode	*Criconemella* spp.
11.	Root-knot nematode	*Meloidogyne* spp.
12.	Sheath nematode	*Hemicycliophora* spp.
13.	Spiral nematode	*Helicotylenchus* spp.
14.	Sting nematode	*Belonolaimus* spp.
15.	Stubby-root nematodes	*Paratrichodorus* spp., *Trichodorus* spp.
16.	Stunt nematode	*Tylenchorhynchus* spp.

17. Rice root nematode — *Hirschmanniella* spp.
18. Burrowing nematode — *Radopholus similis*

Nematode Morphology

Nematode Body

The nematode body is divided into three regions. They are outer body tube or body wall, inner body tube and body cavity or pseudocoelom.

Outer body tube

The outer body tube or body wall includes the cuticle, hypodermis, and somatic muscles (Fig. 2). The body wall protects the nematode from the harsh external environment, serves as the exoskeleton and provides the mechanism for movement of the organism through the soil and plant tissue. The body wall also contains much of the nervous and secretory-excretory systems, and it plays a role in the exchange of gases.

Cuticle or Exoskeleton

The cuticle is a non living, non cellular, triple-layered covering that is secreted by the underlying hypodermis. The cuticle is flexible. It covers the entire body and lines the oesophagus, vulva, anus, cloaca, excretory pore and sensory organs. The feeding stylet and copulatory spicules are formed from cuticle.

The composition and form of the cuticle is highly variable. In general, the cuticle is composed of three primary zones *viz*., the cortical layer, median layer and basal layer.

The cuticle of many nematodes have markings on the surface. They are varied and complex and have been often used by taxonomists to assist in the identification of various species. The cuticular markings are categorised into different types.

i. Punctations
ii. Transverse markings or striations and
iii. Longitudinal markings.

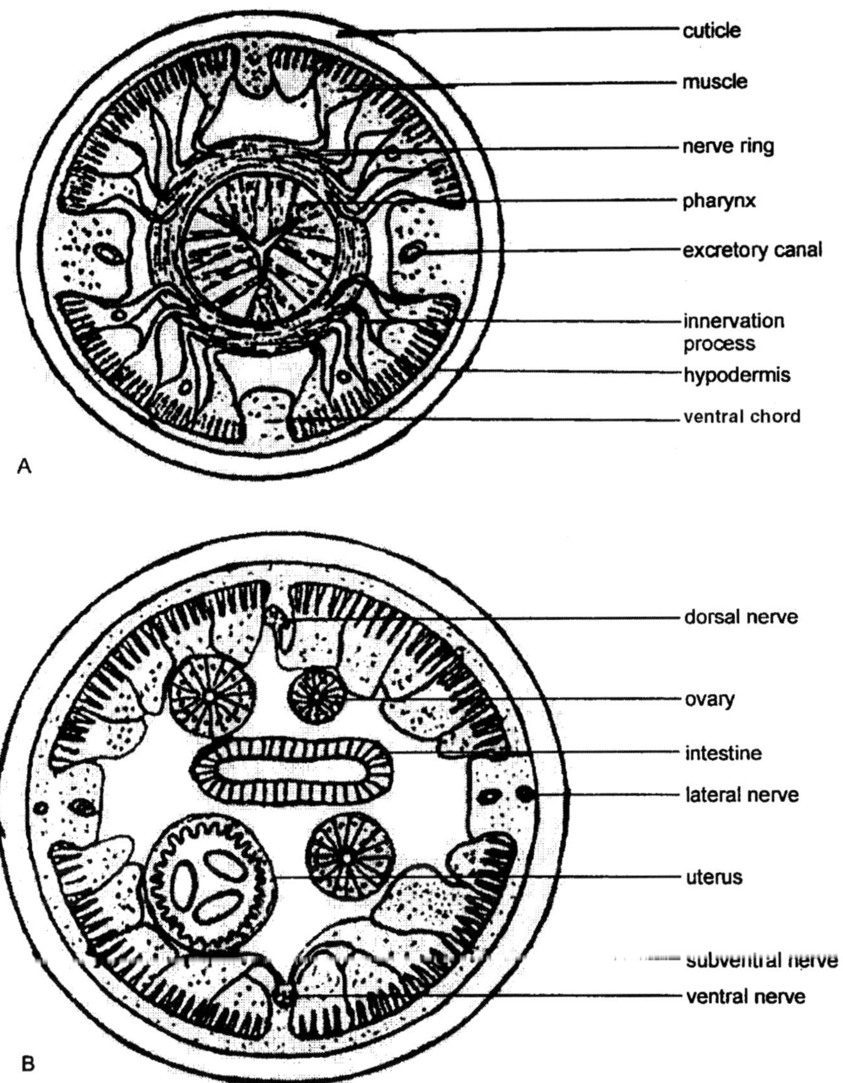

Fig. 2: Transverse sections through the oesophageal region **(A)** and the middle region **(B)** of the nematode

i) *Punctations:* These are minute, round dots arranged in a pattern. They act as structures for strengthening the cuticle rather than pore canals through which cuticular proteins may be transported. In the perineal pattern of *Meloidogyne hapla* these punctations can be seen.

ii) *Transverse markings or Striations:* There are transverse lines present on the surface of the cuticle. These markings exhibit distinct variations among the plant parasitic nematodes and often used by the taxonomists for identification. The transverse markings cause a pattern of ridges and furrows right from head to tail and these markings gives the false appearance as if the nematode is segmented. These markings are well pronounced in some families such as Criconematidae, Tylenchidae and Heteroderidae. In Criconematids, the annulations are clearly visible and known as scales and spines (Fig.3). The perineal pattern in the posterior body region of *Meloidogyne* females as well as rugose wall pattern of *Heterodera* cysts, are considered to be the modifications of transverse markings.

iii) *Longitudinal markings:* These markings are the lines on the cuticle which runs longitudinally throughout the length of the nematode body. These markings are divided into a) lateral lines or incisures and b) longitudinal ridges.

a) *Lateral lines or Incisures:* These are lines running longitudinal to the body axis of nematode but they are confined to the lateral field in area just on top of lateral hypodermal chords on either side of the nematode body running throughout the length. The number of lateral lines or incisures is an important taxonomic character as it shows stability within the genus.

b) *Longitudinal ridges:* Longitudinal ridges are raised lines present on cuticle running longitudinal to nematode body axis but are confined in the area other than lateral field. The number of these ridges is used by taxonomists for species identification.

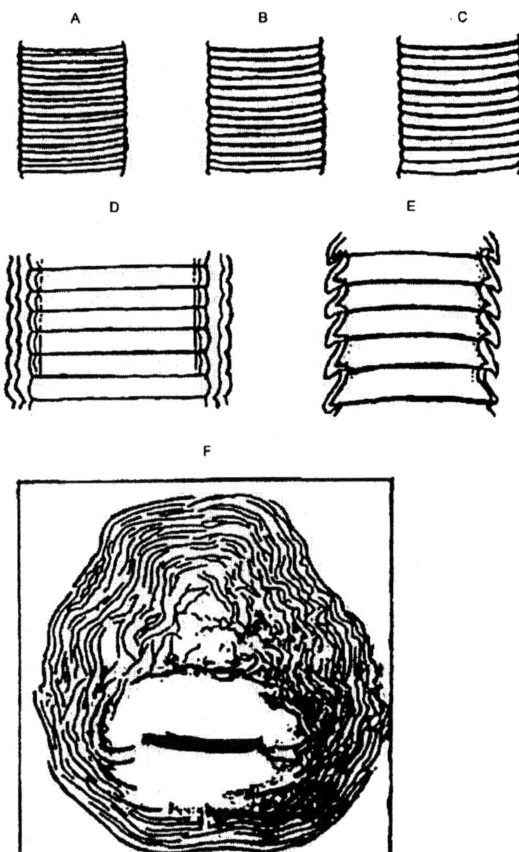

A.Tylenchus, B. Tylenchorhynchus, C. Hoplolaimus
D. Hemicycliophora, E. Criconema and
F. Perineal pattern of Meloidogyne

Fig. 3: Culticular annulation in nematodes

Apart from this, alae are also present. They are thickening or projections of the cuticle which occur in the lateral or sublateral region. There are three types of alae.

i. Caudal alae
ii. Cervical alae and
iii. Longitudinal alae

i) *Caudal alae:* These are found in the posterior region and restricted to males as copulatory bursa.

ii) *Cervical alae:* These are confined to the anterior part of the nematode body. Cervical alae are found in some species of marine nematodes.

iii) *Longitudinal alae:* The longitudinal alae delimit the lateral fields and are known as lateral alae. Their form varies in different species. They are transversed by striations or furrows varying in number from 1 to 12. Functionally, they probably assist in locomotion and may permit slight changes in the width of nematodes.

The functions of cuticle

Cuticle gives definite shape and size to the body, acts as an exoskeleton, helps in movement, being semipermeable, it regulates permeability and provides important taxonomic characters for identification of nematodes.

Cuticular layering

The nematode cuticle consists of three layers *viz.*, an outer layer (cortical layer), a middle layer (median or matrix) and an inner layer (basal or fiber layer). In some nematodes there are only two layers as in the adult females of the family Heteroderidae.

1. Outer layer (Cortical layer)

The cortical layer is amorphous and electron dense layer. In many forms, the cortical layer is divided into an external cortical layer and an internal cortical layer. The surface of the external cortical layer is exposed to the environment. This layer is very thin measuring about 25 to 40 μ and can be subdivided into an outer membrane (3-5 μ thick) and may correspond with a triple layered plasma membrane.

The external cortical layer has been considered to be a keratin. The disulphide group present in this layer is responsible for resistant properties. In cyst nematodes, this layer become highly resistant due to quinone tanning of the cuticle. For example, in potato cyst nematode, *Globodera rostochiensis* and cyst nematode, *Heterodera* spp., the cuticle of the female on maturity becomes tough and leathery to form cyst which protect hundreds of eggs.

The internal cortical layer varies considerably in thickness in different nematodes. In preparasitic juvenile forms it may be about 0.15 to 0.25μ thick. It has a fibrous structure. There is no clear cut demarcation separating the internal cortical layer and median layer. This layer appears to be biochemically active in some nematodes. Enzymes and RNA were detected from this layer.

2. Median layer (Middle layer)

The average thickness of the median layer is 0.1μ in the juveniles of *Meloidogyne* and *Heterodera*. This layer undergoes marked change in the width in *Hemicycliophora arenaria* as it grows to become adult. The median layer in this nematode is about 0.2μ in width in the second stage juvenile and about 0.7μ in width in adult female. Chemically this layer consists of proteins resembling collagen. A non-specific esterase, acid muco-polysaccharide and some lipids have been detected in this layer. It does not appear to be as metabolically active as that of cortical layer.

3. Inner layer (Basal / fibre layer)

The basal or fibre layer consists of regularly arranged vertical rods or striations. It is composed of protein with very close linkage between the molecules, resulting in resistant layer which protect the nematode from environment. The thickness of the basal layer varies from 125-500μ.

Hypodermis

The hypodermis, which can be cellular or partially cellular, secretes the cuticle. It lies beneath the cuticle and contains longitudinal thickening between the somatic muscles that contain the nuclei, mitochondria, lipid droplets, endoplasmic reticulum, longitudinal nerves and the canals of the secretory-excretory system. Most nematodes have four hypodermal chords (one dorsal, one ventral and two lateral chords).

Hypodermal glands

The hypodermal glands vary in different species of nematodes. They act as either osmotic or ionic regulators. The caudal glands of the hypodermis are found in the tail region. The caudal gland (usually 3 to 5 in number) secrets the adhesive substances which help to anchor the nematodes. The hypodermal glands are also associated with the sensory organs like amphids, phasmids and deirids.

Somatic musculature

The somatic muscle cells are arranged in a single layer. The muscle cells are spindle shaped and attached to the hypodermis throughout their length. A non-striated, non-contractile portion of the muscle cell contains the nucleus and other cell organelles.

It is connected to the nervous system by an elongated process of noncontractile portion of the muscle cell. The muscle cells on the ventral side of the nematode body are attached to the ventral nerve and all the cells on the dorsal side are connected to the dorsal nerve. Therefore, stimulation of muscles by the dorsal and ventral nerves causes contractions in the dorso-ventral plane and results in the characteristic sinusoidal movement of the nematode.

Muscle Cells

On the basis of arrangement of muscle cells, the following 3 types are identified.

a) Holomyarian : having two muscle cells in each zone.

b) Meromyarian : 2 or 5 muscle cells in each interchordal zone

c) Polymyarian : More than 5 muscle cells per zone.

On the basis of the muscle cell shape, they are grouped as

a) Platymyarian: A flat type of cell with contractile elements limited in places to the base lying close to the epidermis.

b) Coelomyarian: 'U' shaped cells in which muscle fibre are adjacent and perpendicular to the hypodermis and extend along the sides of the muscle cell of varying distances.

c) Circomyarian: This type of muscle cells are almost round and the muscle fibres completely surround the cytoplasm.

The platymyarian muscle cell is considered primitive which might have modified into coelomyarian type of narrowing and upward elongation of the fibrillar zone. Muscle cells are connected to each other by means of cytoplasmic bridges and have nerve connections.

In addition to somatic muscle, there are many specialized muscles, which are associated with feeding, food movement and defecation (cephalic, oesophageal, intestinal and anal muscles) as well as with reproduction (vulval, spicular, gubernacular, copulatory and bursal muscles).

Inner Body Tube

Digestive system

The nematode digestive system is the inner body tube into which some glands open. The digestive system of nematodes include the stoma, oesophagus, intestine and anus. The inner body tube is divided into 3 main regions.

1. Stomodeum : which constitutes the stoma, oesophagus and cardia.
2. Mesenteron : which constitutes the intestine.
3. Proctodeum : which is the posterior-most region comprising of rectum and anal opening.

1. Stomodeum

Stoma is the portion of the inner body tube lying between the oral opening and oesophagus. It shows high degree of variations depending upon the feeding habits of different genera of nematodes. The stomatal opening is small and slit like and surrounded by an oval-shaped prestoma that is encircled by the small pit-like opening of the six inner labial sensilla. The stomatal opening occurs on the labial disc and is surrounded by six lips (two subdorsal, two subventral and two lateral).

The variation in head, stylet and lip of different nematodes *viz.*, *Tylenchorhynchus*, *Pratylenchus, Helicotylenchus, Hoplolaimus, Radopholus, Aphelenchus, Xiphinema, Mononchus, Aphelenchoides, Hemicycliophora* and *Criconemoides* are furnished in Fig. 4.

Plant parasitic nematodes are armed with a protrusible stylet which is usually hollow and functions like a hypodermic needle. In Secernentea, the stylet is thought to be derived from fusion of the stomatal lining and therefore called as **stomato stylet** (Fig. 4A). The stomato stylet consists of an anterior cone, a cylindrical shaft and three rounded basal knobs. The stylet protractor muscles are attached to the knobs. However, in Adenophorea, the stylet is thought to be derived from a tooth and therefore, it is called as **odonto stylet** (Fig. 4A). The posterior end of the odonto stylet may have an extension and three flanges that serve as points of attachment for the stylet protractor muscles (Fig. 4A).

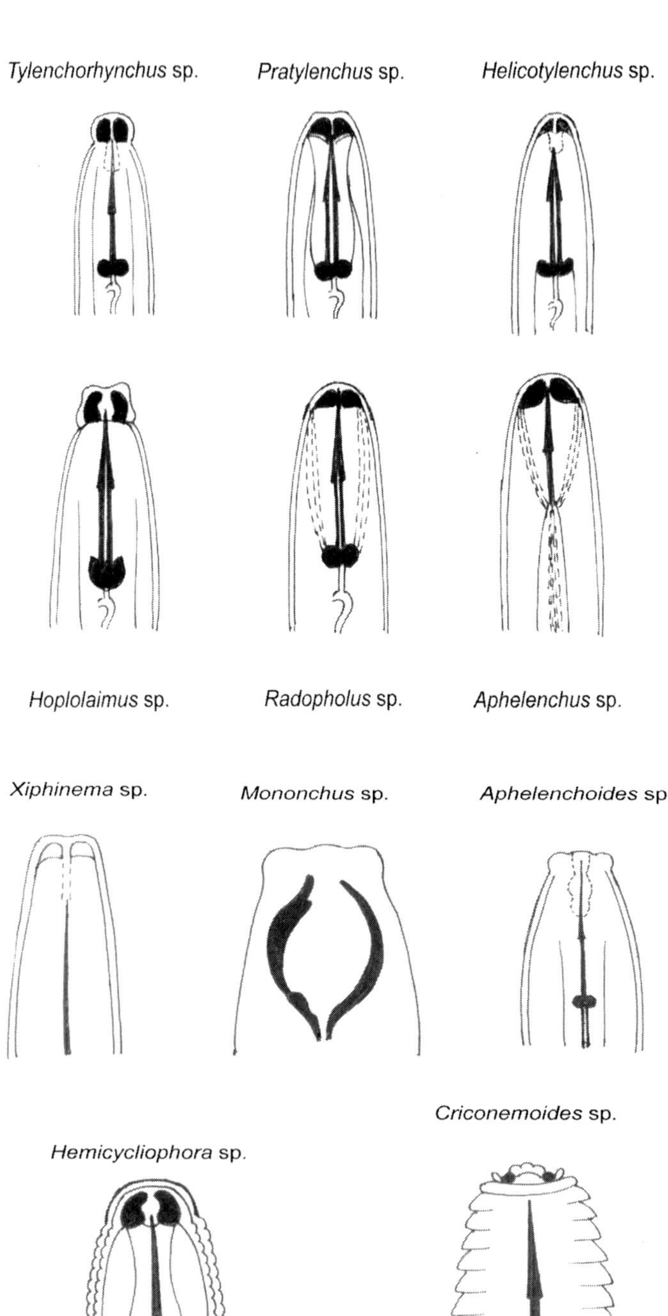

Fig. 4: Variations in head stylet and lip region

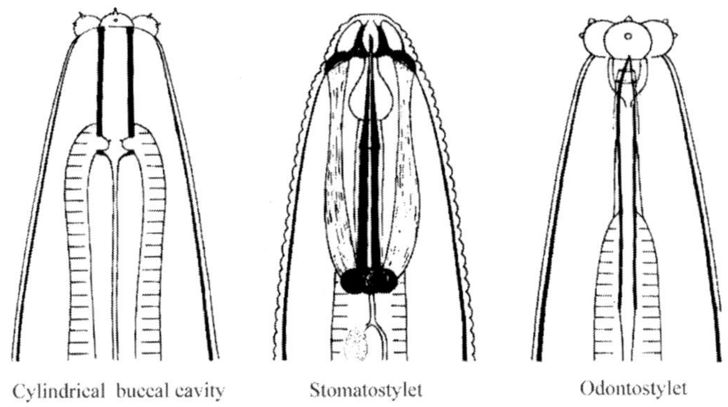

Fig. 4A: Different types of stylets in nematodes

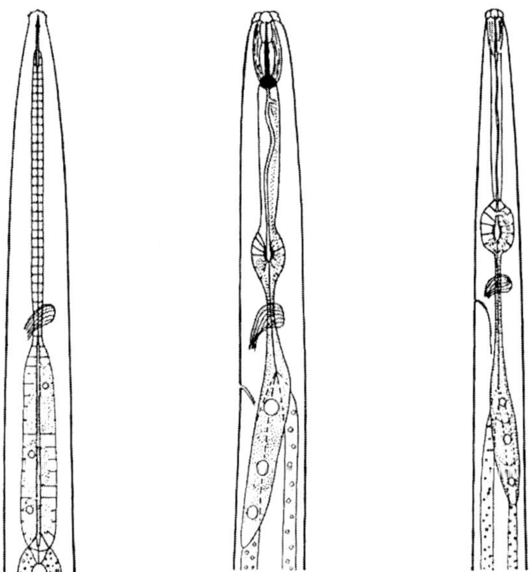

Fig. 4B: Different types of oesophagus in nematodes

In some plant parasitic nematodes like *Trichodorus* and *Paratrichodorus*, the odontostylet is distinctly curved ventrally, lacks flanges and it is solid. It functions to pierce the cell wall of the root. The nematode secretes a hollow tube out of its stoma that connects it with the plant. This feeding tube serves as the interface between the nematode and the plant.

The different types of stylet found in *Pratylenchus, Hoplolaimus, Criconemoides, Xiphinema,* and *Longidorus* are furnished in Fig. 4C.

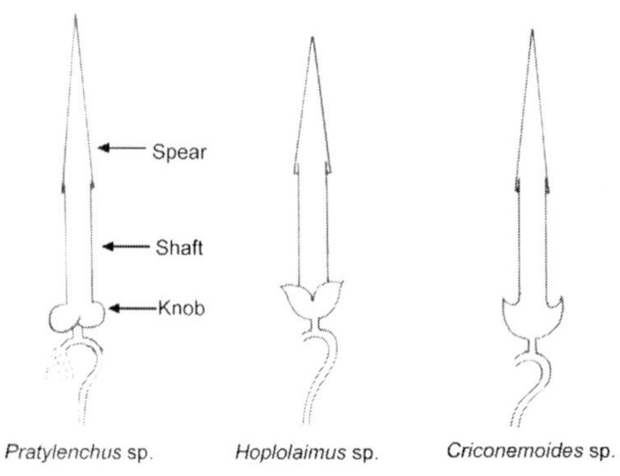

Odonto stylet - Dorylaimids

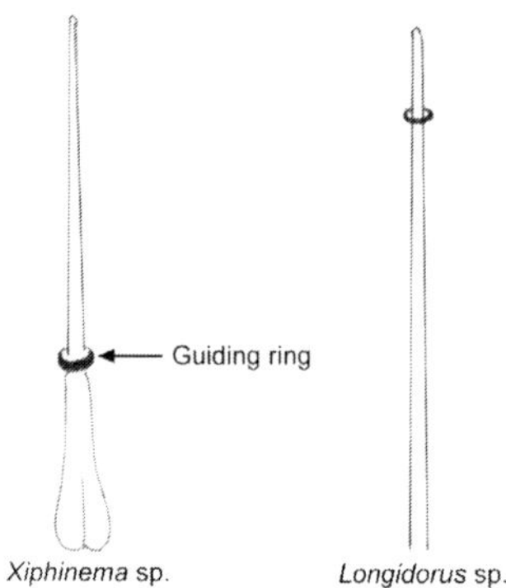

Fig. 4C: Different types of stylet Stomato stylet - Tylenchids

Oesophagus or pharynx

The oesophagus is a muscular pumping organ attached to the posterior portion of the stylet lined with cuticle. In Adenophorea, the oesophagus is divided into a narrow anterior procorpus and a broad posterior corpus. Three or five oesophageal gland cells empty into the lumen (one dorsal and two to four subventral in position). However, in Secernentea the oesophagus is divided into distinct regions, such as narrow procorpus, followed by a broad muscular median bulb or pump, a narrow isthmus and a gland lobe. The gland lobe may overlap the intestine in some genera and contain three to six gland cells (one dorsal and two sub-ventral). In the order Tylenchida, it empties within the median bulb. The oesophagus has valve (cordia) at the posterior end which prevent the regurgitation of food. The three types of oesophagus *viz*., Dorylaimoid, Tylenchoid and Aphelenchoid are furnished in Fig. 4B.

2. Mesenteron or intestine

The nematode intestine is a simple, hollow, straight tube consisting of a single layer of epithelial cells. The intestine is generally divided into three regions which merge into each other without any perceptible boundaries. They are the anterior or ventricular region, the midintestinal region and the posterior or prerectal region. The **microvilli** are finger like projections of the plasma membrane projecting into the intestinal region. They increase the surface area of the intestine and are both secretory and absorbtive in function. Each intestinal cell is surrounded by a plasma membrane and whole intestine is separated from the pseducoelom by a basement membrane. The intestinal cells are rich in glycogen, lamellar bodies, large protein and lipid or fat bodies. These make up the storage material in the infective juveniles of many parasitic nematodes. The food moves in the intestine by the ingestion of more food and also by locomotory activity of the nematode.

3. Proctodeum

Proctodeum comprises rectum and anus. The intestinal tube is connected with a narrow small tube at the posterior end, through a valve or sphincter muscles known as rectum. It regulates the flow of undigested food material which is to be passed outside the nematode body through a ventrally located aperture known as anus.

The opening and closing of anus is governed by certain specialised muscles attached with it. In male nematode, the rectum joins with the hind part of the testis forming a common opening known as cloaca. In female, there is a separate opening.

Tail comprises the region from anal opening to tail tip. Among the invertebrates the tail is unique to nematodes. The tail is absent in adult females of root knot and cyst nematodes. The tail are of different shapes *viz.*, filiform, fusiform, conoid, dorsally convex, arcuate, mucronate tail, digitate etc., are furnished in Fig. 4D.

Glands

Oesophageal and rectal glands are present in nematodes. The oesophageal gland enter the stomodeum and rectal gland enter proctodeum.

Oesophageal glands

Three uninucleated oesophageal glands are present. One gland on dorsal and other two ventro lateral or sub ventral in position. These glands connect with the lumen of the oesophagus by means of ducts, often by means of a terminal swelling or ampulla.

The oesophageal glands have been thoroughly studied in *Meloidogyne* and they have important role in hatching, host penetration and also establishment of host parasitic relationship.

Rectal glands

The rectal gland number varies in different species and between male and female of the same species. These glands are responsible for the copious production of gelatinous mucopolysaccharide matrix in which eggs are deposited as a mass (eg. *Meloidogyne*). It protects the eggs from adverse environmental conditions.

Function of digestive system

Digestive juices which is secreted from dorsal oesophageal glands are injected into the host plant cell by means of the stylet. During feeding, a distinct zone develop around the feeding site in the host cell. There are two feeding phases.

1. Injection phase or salivation phase, 2. Ingestion phase

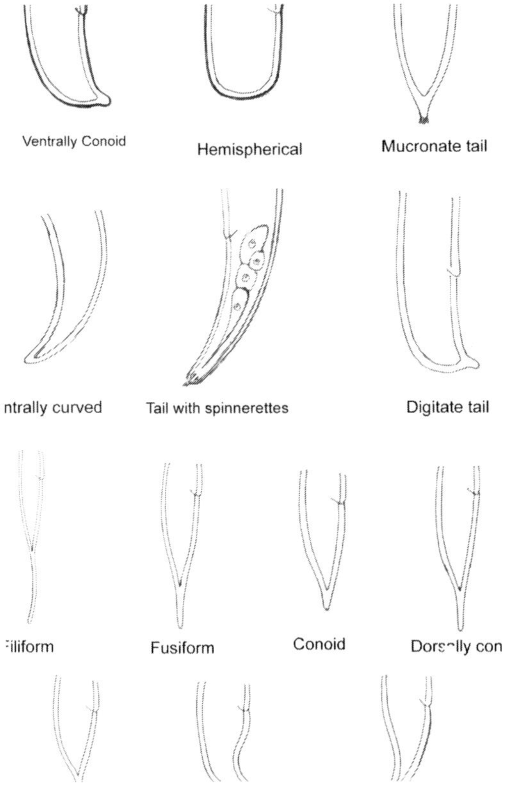

Fig. 4D: Tail Shapes

Injection phase or salivation phase

During this phase, the flow of salivary juices into the host cell occurs due to contraction of lateral muscle of the median bulb.

Ingestion phase

During this phase, rhythmical contraction of the posterior part of the oesophagus associated with the median bulb occurs and in some forms, the oesophageo-intestinal valve or cardia is responsible for ingestion of material from the host.

Various glands associated with the digestive system play an important role in secretion. The cells of these glands are associated with protein and mucopolysaccharide synthesis and their products are shed through cuticle lined ducts either into stomodeum or proctodeum.

The intestine acts as an excretory organ and defecation is mechanically controlled and it is an intense process.

Reproductive system

The nematodes are generally dioecious. Majority of plant parasitic nematodes do not exhibit any differences as far as body shape. Both sexes are vermiform. However, sexual dimorphism is observed in some genera *viz., Meloidogyne, Heterodera, Globodera, Rotylenchulus, Tylenchulus* and *Nacobbus.* The females of these genera become enlarged and assume different shapes after attaining maturity.

Female Reproductive system

The female reproductive system (Fig. 5A) comprises a tube at the top of which the tubular ovary is located. The foremost part of the ovary, where production of ova takes place is known as growth zone followed by maturation zone where further development of eggs takes place. It is followed by a pouch-like structure known as spermatheca where sperms are stored or retained. It is followed by a muscular structure known as quadricolumella which is followed by comparatively broader muscular structure known as uterus. The extension of uterus beyond vulval opening is known as post-vulval uterine sac which may be absent in certain nematode genera, but is mostly present in nematodes having single ovary as observed in the genera *Pratylenchus* and *Ditylenchus*. The uterus opens outside to a ventrally located vulval opening through a tube known as vagina which is a cuticularised structure.

The female reproductive system shows variations within plant parasitic nematodes (Fig.6). Since these structures make a constant character, they are successfully utilised for identification of nematodes. In plant parasitic nematodes the number of ovary may be one or two. When there is one ovary that condition is known as **monodelphic** and when the number is two, the condition is called as **didelphic.**

In monodelphic condition, the ovary is always, anteriorly directed, i.e. **Prodelphic**. In case of didelphic ovaries, if both the ovaries are anteriorly directed and vulva is terminal in position then the condition is known as **didelphic prodelphic** as found in the cáse of *Meloidogyne, Heterodera* and *Globodera.* In some nematodes, two ovaries are opposite to one another, such that one is anteriorly directed and the other posteriorly directed. This is called as **didelphic amphidelphic** condition, as found in the case of *Tylenchorhynchus, Hoplolaimus*, *Helicotylenchus* and *Radopholus.*

In Monodelphic condition, the single ovary is anteriorly directed as in the case of *Ditylenchus* and *Pratylenchus*. It may or may not possess post-vulval uterine sac. In *Agelenchus* and *Zanenthus*, single anteriorly directed ovary is seen which is without post-vulval uterine sac. In such case the vagina is curved. In *Coslenchus* post vulval uterine sac is present with vagina right angled to body axis. In *Cosaglenchus,* the vagina is curved and post vulval uterine sac is present. Its presence may be equal or slightly more than the corresponding body width. In *Aphelenchus*, it is more than double the corresponding width. The vulval opening is a transverse slit and not covered with any flap, but in *Agelenchus* and *Coslenchus* vulva is covered with membranous flap known as vulval flap. The vaginal tube in *Hoplolaimus* and *Cosaglenchus* are provided with a cuticular sclerotised structure encircling the tube known as epiptygma.

The ovary is provided with a double row of cells arranged throughout the length in majority of plant parasitic nematodes. However, in *Anguina,* there are multiple rows of cells arranged linearly. Ovary in most of the plant parasitic nematodes is always straight and does not curve back. Such ovaries are called as **outstretched ovaries** as in the case of *Tylenchorhynchus, Radopholus* and *Hirschmanniella.* In Dorylaimids, the tip of the ovary is curved back. It is known as **reflexed ovary**.

If the ovary is single and posteriorly directed, then it is known as **monodelphic ophisthodelphic** condition and such conditions are rarely seen (eg. *Xiphinema* spp.).

Whenever a nematode has a single ovary, the vulva is posteriorly located to the mid-body region. In majority of nematodes which have two ovaries with amphidelphic condition, the position of vulva is median. Further, an ovary is called **hologenic** if it produced oocytes throughout its length and **telogenic** if producing oocytes only at its distal end.

Male Reproductive System

It comprises a cylindrical tube known as testis which opens along with the digestive tract in a common opening known as **cloaca**. The testis is differentiated into (i) Seminal vesicle, (ii) Vas deferens and (iii) Testis proper (Fig. 5B).

The production of sperms takes place in testis. In nematodes, whenever the number of testis is one, it is known as **monorchic** condition and when they are two in number, the condition is known as **diorchic**. The cloacal region is followed by a protrusible spicule which moves forward and backward with help of specialised muscles attached with its head region. Spicule is narrower at its tip. A cuticularised structure lying beneath the pair of spicule is known as **gubernaculum** which helps and gives support in movement of the spicule. At the tail end, two filamentous cuticular expansions are found and they are known as **bursa or caudal alae**. The bursa helps to hold the female during copulation. Plant parasitic nematodes can reproduce sexually where male and female couplate and give rise to off-springs. Sexual reproduction is also called as **amphimictic** reproduction. **Parthenogenetic** reproduction is also common phenomenon in *Meloidogyne* and *Tylenchulus semipenetrans.*

Sex reversal

In root-knot nematodes (*Meloidogyne* spp.) sometimes sex reversal takes place. This happens during stress period, when there is scarcity of food and also due to unfavourable conditions. Under stress conditions the developing females get converted into males.

Inter sexes

In general like *Meloidogyne* and *Ditylenchus* inter sexes are found. In such cases one reproductive system act as male gonad and other one as female gonad.

Excretory System

The excretory system is not well developed in nematodes. The excretory pore is located in the anterior midventral line close to the **nerve ring**. The position of excretory pore may vary in different genera and even in different stages of the same species. In *T. semipenetrns* the excretory pore is located in the posterior region and its function is rather secretory than excretory. It secrets gelatinous matrix.

The excretory system in nematodes are of two types.

1. Glandular type
2. Tubular type (Fig. 7)

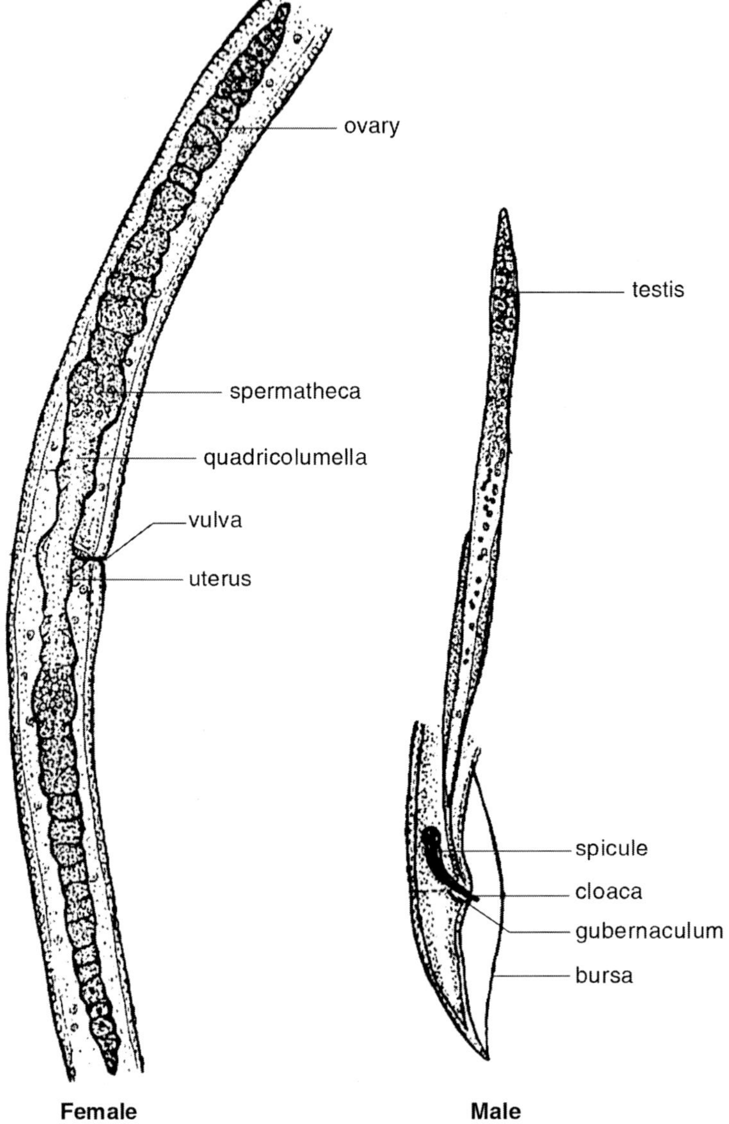

Fig. 5: Reproductive system

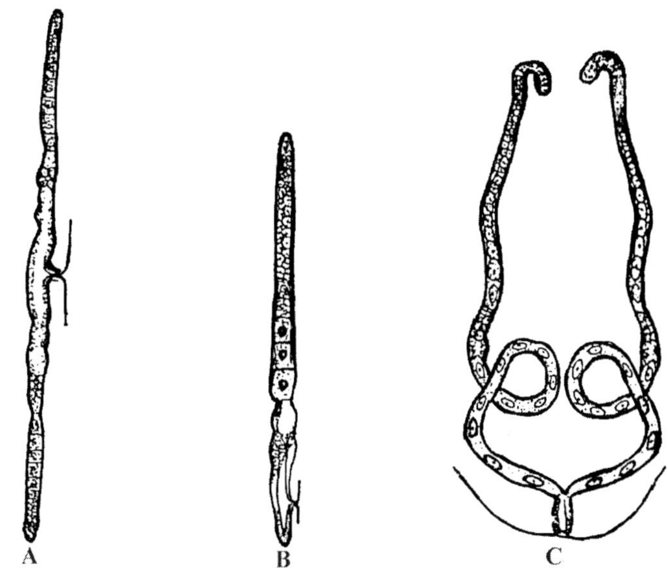

A - Didelphic (Tylenchorhynchus) **B** - Monodelphic (Ditylenchus)
C - Didelphic and prodelphic (Meloidogyne)

Fig. 6: Different types of ovaries in female nematode

Glandular type

The glandular type consists of a single specialised cell known as **renette cell**. It has a posteriorly located enlarged gland known as excretory gland or ventral gland. This gland is connected to the excretory pore by a duct that terminates in a pouch like structure known as ampulla. This type is found in members of the class Adenophorea.

Tubular type

The tubular type of excretory system consists of four-cuticularised canals. Two are anterior and another two are posterior canals. There is a pouch like structure in the middle which connects both the lateral canals. It is known as excretory pore. There are four types in tubular system.

1. Asymmerical or Tylenchid type
2. Inverted 'U' shaped or Ascarid type
3. Rhabditid type
4. Simple 'H' shaped or Oxyurid type

Asymmetrical or Tylenchid type : Majority of the plant parasitic nematodes which fall under the order Tylenchida have this asymmetrical tubular type excretory system. In this type a single tube runs throughout the nematode body length and found in either of the lateral hypodermal chords. In the middle of the single canal, the lumen enlarges to form excretory sinus which is a nucleated structure. It opens through the anterior canal by separating as a small branch tube.

Inverted 'U' shaped or Ascarid type : In this type three canals are found. Out of the three canals, one is located anteriorly and two are located posteriorly. The anterior canal opens outside through an excretory pore located at its tip.

Rhabditid type : Four cuticularised canals are present. Two are located anteriorly and another two are posterior in position. Excretory sinus is modified into two excretory gland in between lateral canals. These glands open ventrally as excretory pore.

Simple 'H' shaped type : This type has four tubular cuticularised canals. Two canals are anterior and slightly shorter than the two canals located posteriorly. These canals are connected by a swollen excretory sinus which opens externally as excretory pore. This type of tubular excretory system is commonly observed in the members of the order Oxyurida. This is a very primitive type of excretory system in nematodes.

Functions of excretory system

1. Excretion of toxic substances.
2. Secretion of certain chemicals.
3. Osmoregulation.
4. In *T. semipenetrans*, excretory pore secretes gelatinous matrix which bind and protect the eggs from abnormal environmental conditions.

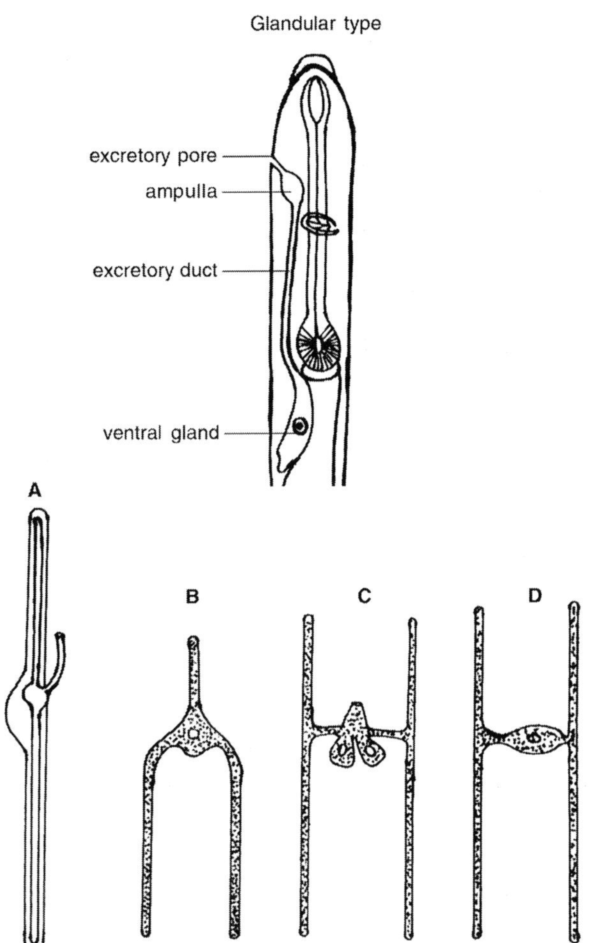

A - Tylenchid type **B** - Ascarid type **C** - Rhabditid type **D** - Oxyurid type

Fig. 7: Different types of excretory system in nematodes

Nervous System

In plant parasitic nematodes, the nervous system is not well developed. Though they possess very primitive type of nervous system, they also respond to different stimuli.

The nervous system in plant parasitic nematodes is of two types

1. Peripheral Nervous System
2. Central Nervous System

Peripheral Nervous System

In plant parasitic nematodes, it is located in the periphery which mainly includes body cuticle and also the cephalic and caudal regions. The parts of nervous system located are well connected with the **nerve ring** (circum oesophageal commissure) which encircles the isthmus region of oesophagus and are considered to be the most important part of the nervous system (brain of nematode). The peripheral nervous system includes the sensory organs such as **cephalic papillae, amphids, cephalids, hemizonid, hemizonions, deirids, phasmids and caudalids.**

Cephalic papillae

These are located on the cephalic region and are 16 in number, two each in two sub-dorsal lips and sub-ventral lips; one each in two lateral lips in outer circle; and one each in all the six lips in inner circle. These papillae are supplied with neurons or nerve fibres arising from the nerve ring. The papillae act as chemoreceptors. They are believed to take part in movement of nematode, governing directions and also in differentiating between host and non-host plants.

Amphids

A pair of amphids is located on both the lateral sides. The amphidial opening in plant parasitic nematodes is located on each lateral lip. The position and opening of amphids is an important diagnostic character in differentiating Tylenchids from other groups. In plant parasitic nematodes, the amphidial opening is pore-like and labial in position, whereas, in Dorylaimids and certain other groups, it is post-labial and may be of different types (Fig. 8). The amphids are also connected with the nerve ring, hence they are sensory in nature. In dorylaimid nematodes and other free living forms the amphids are much more developed as compared to those in parasitic forms. In dorylaimid and free living nematodes, the amphidial opening shows modification and they are not always remaining pore like as in the case or Tylenchids. In Chromodorids, the amphidial opening is spiral, while it is loop-like in *Axnolaimus*. In Plectids, it is question mark shaped whereas in Monhysterids it is circular. In Dorylaimids and Enoplids, cyathiform-shaped opening is seen. In all these cases, the opening is post-labial in position. In Tylenchids, the amphidial aperture is pore-like but in *Psilenchus, Basiria* and *Tylodorus* the opening is slit-like.

Cephalids

These are found in cephalic region. They are sensory structures forming a bend which encircles the nematode body. A pair of cephalids is found, of which one is anterior and other is posterior in position. The exact functions of cephalids are not known. It is believed that they take part in transmitting message to the centrally located nerve ring.

Hemizonid and Hemizonion

They are also supplied with nerve fibres from the nervous system. They are epidermal in origin. They are highly refractive, biconvex, semicircular and may be anterior or posterior to the excretory pore. They form ventro-lateral commissures connecting nerve ring to ventral nerve chord located between cuticle and hypodermis. Hemizonid is anterior to the excretory pore.

Hemizonions are smaller than Hemizonids and are located posterior to hemizonid, forming a small ventro-lateral commissure. Hemizonion is not always present unlike hemizonids. Hemizonid and hemizoninon are believed to be involved in neurosecretion.

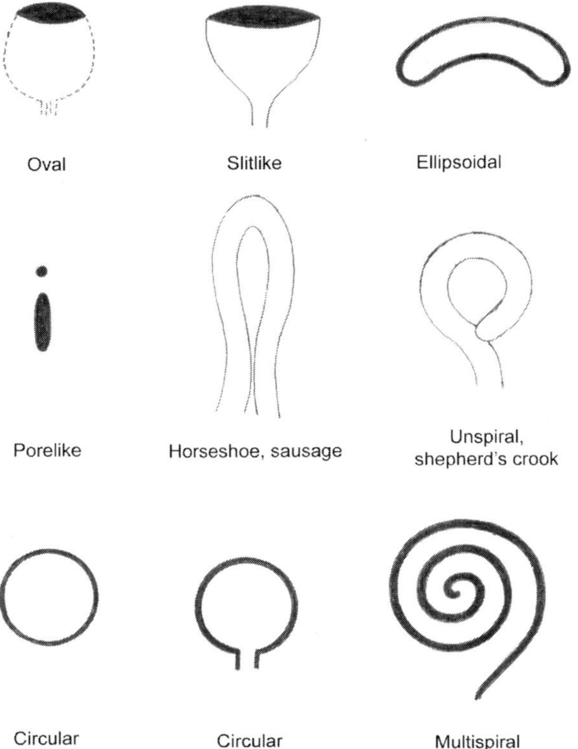

Fig. 8: Amphid Shapes

Deirids

These are a pair of small protruberance, one each in lateral side in the middle of the lateral field. These are located in the region of oesophagus at the region of excretory pore. These are always present in members of family Tylenchidae and Neotylenchidae while absent in members of subfamily Tylenchorhynchinae, Criconematinae and Dolichodorinae. They are also sensory organs, which do not have exterior opening like amphids and phasmids. Since these are not present in all plant parasitic nematodes, it is believed that they have no definite role to play and their presence is not essentially required.

Phasmids

Phasmids are also sensory organs located in the posterior half of the nematode, paired, one each in lateral side of nematode and present in middle of lateral field. They open outside through a minute pore. The presence and absence of phasmids is of immense diagnostic value in differentiating **Phasmida** (**having phasmids**) from **Aphasmida (not having phasmids).** In certain Tylenchids e.g. *Aphasmatylenchus* and members of superfamily Criconematoidea, phasmids are absent. In case of sub family Hopolaiminae, phasmids are comparatively more prominent. When size of phasmids are bigger then these are called as **scutella**. They are present in *Scutellonema*. Main functions of phasmids are chemoreception, mechanoreception and thermoreception.

Caudalids

Caudalids are present in front of the tail representing anolumbar commissure joining pre-anal ganglion to lumbar ganglion. Definite function of caudalids are not known. It is believed that they may take part in transmitting message from tail to the nerve ring.

Central Nervous System

Central nervous system comprises the nerve ring which is a band of nerve fibres. It encircles isthmus. Nerve ring governs various functions of the nematode body. A few species of nematodes are known to have two nerve rings. Associated with this nerve ring are a small dorsal ganglion, two or more lateral ganglion and a ventral ganglion, which is sometimes divided into two. Six or eight longitudinal nerves run posteriorly from these ganglion. Six nerves pass forward from the nerve ring and supply the lips and associated sense organs. The ventral nerve which runs in the ventral chord is the largest nerve and is a paired structure for some of its length. The dorsal nerve which originate from the dorsal ganglion runs in the dorsal chord is much smaller.

A small nerve which arises from the lateral ganglion runs posteriorly along each lateral chord and in many nematodes sub-dorsal and sub-ventral nerves are also present. The dorsal and lateral nerves have a few ganglion associated with them but the ventral nerve has several ganglion along its length. Several commissures, running in the hypodermis, connect the longitudinal nerves at regular intervals along the length of the nematode (Fig. 8).

A pair of nerves runs forward from the lateral ganglion to the amphids at the anterior end of the nematode. The dorsal nerve is said to be chiefly motor and lateral nerves mainly sensory in function. The sub-median and the ventral nerves are partly motor and partly sensory. There is a system of three nerves in the pharynx, one in each sector, which are connected with one another by commissures and also with nerve ring. Nematodes are unique in that the muscle cells of the body are innervated by processes which pass from the muscle. It is claimed that the nerve muscle junction is similar to those found in other animals.

Transmission along nerves

Nothing is known about the processes involved in the conduction of an impulse along nerves in nematodes. In *Ascaris*, it is known that the pseudocoelomic fluid contains more sodium as compared with potassium ions. It is thus possible to speculate that the nerve axons in this species function as that of other animals in which the action current arises from an influx of external sodium ions.

Acetylcholine is apparently involved in nervous transmission in nematodes. Acetylcholine like substances have been detected in *Ascaris*. The head region of *Ascaris* was found to contain fifteen times more acetylcholine than that of the remaining body. Cholinesterase activity is observed to be more in the nerve ring, amphids, phasmids and other sense organs in nematodes.

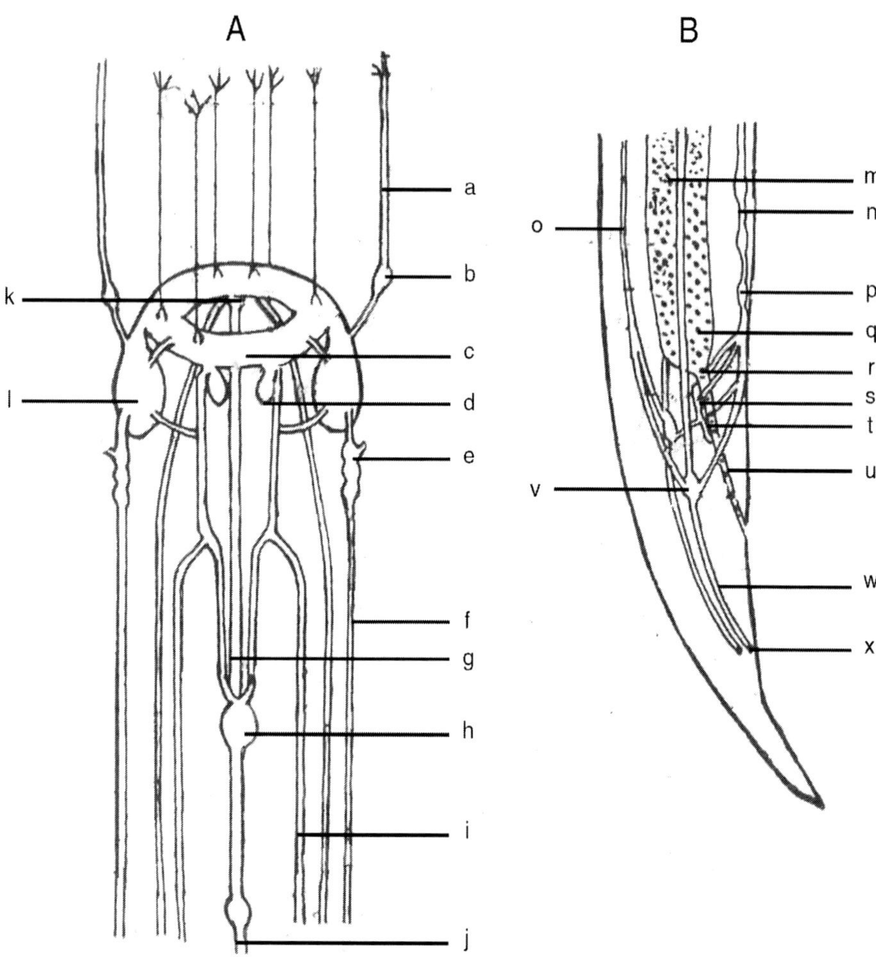

(a) amphidial nerve (b) amphidial ganglion (c) nerve ring (d) ventral ganglion (e) cervical papilla nerve (f) lateral nerve (g) dorsal nerve (h) retrovesicular ganglion (i) latero ventral nerve (j) ventral nerve (k) dorsal ganglion (l) amphid (m) lateral nerve (n) ventral nerve (o) dorsal nerve (p) preanal ganlion (q) intestine (r) rectal commisure (s) dorso rectal ganglion (t) ventro lateral connective (u) rectum (v) lumbar ganglion (w) caudal nerve (x) phasmid

Fig. 8A : Nervous system in anterior region B : Posterior region

4

Biology of Plant Parasitic Nematodes

Life cycle of nematode has six stages. The egg stage, first stage juvenile (J_1), second stage juvenile (J_2), third stage juvenile (J_3), fourth stage juvenile (J_4) and the adult stage.

The first four stages are the immature stages and are known as juvenile stages. The female lays eggs in soil or in plant tissues, singly or in groups as egg mass that hatch out into juveniles which are almost similar to adults appearance. The first moult occurs within the egg shell and the second stage juvenile comes out by rupturing the egg shells as J_2. In case of *Xiphinema index*, the juveniles are reported to emerge from the egg before the first moult. The juvenile cuticle is shed after each moult.

The egg

The nematode eggs are oval in shape. The eggs are covered by three membranes, the external protein layer which is the secretion of uterus wall, the middle chitinous layer or the true shell secreted by egg itself and the inner lipid layer (vitelline layer). The chitin content in the egg shell vary in different species of nematodes.

Embryonic development

The adult female lays the eggs. The egg starts dividing by cleavage of their protoplasms to form cells. The first cleavage occur transverse to the longitudinal axis and gives two equal cells or blastomeres which are the first somatic (S_1) cell and the parental germinal cell (P_1). The second cleavage results in four cells which are first arranged in a T shape. This shape is achieved by the blastomere S_1 dividing longitudinally and the blastomere P1 dividing transversely by P2 and S_2. At last these cells get arranged in a rhomboidal shape. The transverse and longitudinal mitotic divisions of daughter cell continue. The S_1 blastomere is the primary somatic cell and its two products (A&B) produce most of the nematode's ectodermal cells. The S2 blastomere produces somatic tissue and give rise to ectoderm (E), mesoderm (M) and stomodeum (St) tissues. The gonads of nematode are derived from P_1. In the blastula stage the cells are so arranged as to form a fluid filled sphere bound by a single layer of the cells, while in the gastrula stage, the early embryo consists of an open mouthed sac-like body with a wall of two layers of cells (Fig. 9).

The cells A and B further divide to produce a, b, and P_2 divides to give P_3 and S3. The dorsal cells produced by A and B continue to divide and finally give rise to most of the hypodermis, excretory cells and nervous system. The daughter cell P_2 divides into P_4 and S_4. These S_3 and S_4 are ectodermal and produce the hypodermis in the posterior region of the nematode body.

The endodermal tissue produced from the products of cell E_1 and P_1 divides into P_5 and S_5. The descendants of S_5 give covers to the gonads and their ducts, while the products of P_5, G_1, G_2 and their descendants proliferate into germ cells only.

The primary mesodermal cell M gives rise the nematode's body wall musculature and its pseudocoelomic cells, while the pharynx from St cells. During early embryonic stages, these primary cells, St, M and E present on the ventral surface of the embryo and are taken within the embryo by process of gastrulation. In further development the dorso-ventrally flattened embryo is changed to a cylindrical shape. The embryo starts to become worm-shaped and a coiled juvenile is recognised inside the egg membrane. At last, the cell constancy is reached and further cell multiplication stops in all organs except the reproductive system. The first moult takes place within the egg and J_2 ruptures the egg shell and hatch out. Before hatching, the J_1 can be seen riggling inside the egg shell.

The post embryonic development in plant parasitic nematodes takes place within the egg leading to the formation of juvenile which is ready to undergo first moult. In the process of post embryonic development, hatching and moulting are the important stages.

Hatching (Ecdysis)

The term hatching is used for the emergence of the juvenile from the egg. It occurs either in response of a stimulus or stimuli from the host or takes place under normal environment. In cyst forming nematodes, the release of juvenile from cysts is an emergence and not hatching. Eggs have hatched within the cyst. The eggs of *Globodera rostochiensis* generally hatch in response to root exudates (stimuli) provided by Solanaceous crops *viz.,* potato and tomato. After embryonic development the first stage juvenile undergoes the first moult within the egg and thus second stage juveniles are found within the egg. After reaching a particular stage of growth and favourable hatching conditions are present, the juvenile shows vigorous movement, often causing bulging of the egg membrane as seen in case of *Pratylenchus, Paratylenchus, Nacobbus* and *Meloidogyne*. After that the juvenile makes a series of thrusts with the help of stylet on the egg shell @ 40-90 per minute and finally juvenile emerge out by breaking the egg shell at perforated places.

Moulting (Eclosion)

The hatched juvenile resembles the adult except for body size and gonad development. The juvenile undergoes some changes in form, particularly at the anterior and posterior ends and formation of gonads. Growth in nematodes is associated with moulting which usually occurs four times and there are five stages. After the fourth moult, the nematode becomes fully grown adult. During moulting, the entire cuticle, including the cuticular lining of the stoma, stylet, oesophagus, vulva, cloaca, rectum, amphids, phasmids and excretory pore are shed. In most of the plant parasitic nematodes greatest growth occurs after the last moult and moulting tends to occur in the earlier half of the growth curve.

Stimulus

It is reported that the neurosecretory cells of nematodes are stimulated to produce some secretions which activate glands that produce enzymes or hormones which initiate moulting. In some cases root exudates act as stimulus for moulting as in the case of *Paratylenchus nanus* and it acts as a stimulus to the fourth stage juvenile moult. In endoparasitic nematodes, the stimulus may be more complex and may be closely associated with a increase in size of nematode, because in these nematodes moulting does not occur until some growth has completed within the host. The stimulus may depend on the host, temperature, pH and the salt content of the soil. When these factors are optimal, the stimulus acts after a short exposure. Juvenile once stimulated, it releases the exsheathing fluid into space between the new and old cuticle which then digest the area of the sheath near the excretory pore ultimately releasing the juvenile.

The receptor

In all cases, the receptor may be cuticular and hypodermal structure e.g. hemizonid. It seems to be associated with neuro secretory activity which leads to the production of an enzyme which is responsible for moulting.

The juvenile becomes sluggish, inactive and feed vigorously just before moulting. The old cuticle is discarded by abrasion against soil particles or any rough material. The cuticle may be shed in one piece or the anterior part may be shed separately as a cap.

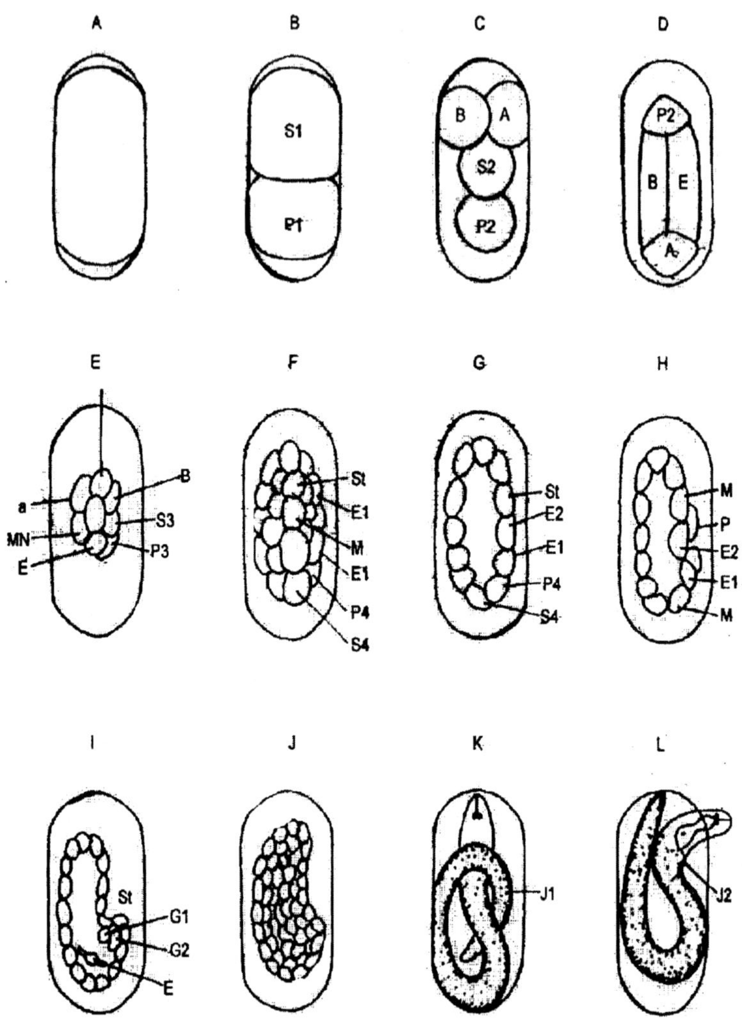

Fig. 9: Nematode embryogenesis

Growth and development

In plant parasitic nematodes, there are four juvenile stages and an adult stage. The immature stage of nematodes are called as juvenile. In case of endoparasitic nematodes, three moults occur within the host plant. The duration of the different juvenile stages is highly variable. Gonad development starts in the first juvenile stage before hatching but the growth of the organs is slow. The development starts with the formation of genital primordia which consist of two control germinal cells or one large cell which are bordered by two smaller somatic cells. External environment affect the structural development and physiology of the host which may influence the development of the nematode. The plant parasitic nematode fixes its feeding site in different regions of the root. *Meloidogyne* goes even up to stelar region, *Heterodera* and *R.reniformis* mostly confine to pericycle and *T.semipenetrans* penetrates cortex region (Fig. 12B).

Life cycle

Root-knot nematodes (*Meloidogyne* spp.)

The root-knot nematodes are sedentary endoparasites of underground plant parts. The eggs are retained in a gelantinous matrix, which normally protrudes out of the host tissues. About 200 to 300 oval eggs are found in a single egg mass which makes its size larger than the female body.

The life cycle starts from the egg usually in the one celled stage deposited by the female. Development of the embryo starts within an hour of deposition, resulting in two, four, eight cells, etc. The embryo and the first stage juvenile move within the egg but not very active.

After the first moult, the second stage infective juvenile is formed within the egg. Juvenile hatch occurs under suitable physical condition but not depending on host root exudate or hatching factor. The emerging second stage juveniles are found free in the soil. They attack new host root tissue in the region behind the root tip (meristamatic zone) (Fig. 10A). The juveniles which develop into females establish feeding site in the pericycle region and become sedentary. Subsequently three moults occur and the juvenile develop into females with spherical body embedded in the host tissue. The neck region is unaltered.

During feeding, the juvenile pierce the cell wall with secretions cause enlargement of cells in the vascular cylinder and increased cell division in the pericycle. The nematode feeding stimulates the development of a typical nurse cell system called **'Syncytium'** or **Giant cell'**. These cells are multinucleate which contain dense cytoplasm and enlarged nuclei with several mitochondrial and golgi bodies and are metabolically active.

The juveniles which develop into adult males are initially parasitic. After moulting three times they leave the host as a worm like form and come closer to the females for copulation. Parthenogenesis is reported to be common in *Meloidogyne*. For development of a mature female it takes around 30 days which may vary depending upon the species of the host and parasite and environmental factors like temperature and soil type.

Cyst nematodes (*Globodera* spp. and *Heterodera* spp.)

Second stage juveniles usually penetrate the root just behind the growing point. These juveniles grow rapidly and three moults occur in the host. In about 5-6 weeks after penetration, the white cysts are clearly visible which protrude from the root surface (Fig. 10B). These young cysts are packed with eggs and upon death the body wall hardens due to quinone tanning into a tough resistant brown covering known as **cysts** and contain viable eggs. The cysts get separated from the root and fall into soil.

Juveniles emergence from cysts is often in response to root exudates from a host plant. The best emergence of juveniles occurs as a result of a rise in temperature after a period of low temperature. Maximum emergence of juveniles from cysts under Indian condition takes place at a temperature of 20-22°C. The cysts continue to release eggs over a period of 3-4 years at the rate of 50 per cent viable eggs per year. There is only one generation of the nematode in a year.

Multiplication of nematode is favoured by soil texture. Migration of second stage juveniles is favoured by light textured soils. The host cells close to the head region of the sedentary female begin to modify and finally enlarge to form multinucleate syncytium with a thick outer boundary. The female feeds from this nurse cell system and grows. The swollen adult female protrudes out of the root tissues and later changes into brown cysts.

Although cyst nematodes induce giant cell formation, gall formation is not distinct. Each syncytium is associated with only one nematode in the case of cyst nematodes unlike the root-knot nematodes where one or more nematodes are associated with a syncytium. Nuclei is enlarged in the syncytium caused by the root-knot nematode but in cyst nematode nuclei is relatively small. The syncytia are bound by the vascular elements especially xylem which develops specific wall ingrowths. There is a enlarged nucleoli and irregular nuclei. Abundant mitochondria, golgi bodies, protoplasts and dense endoplasmic reticula are also found in the syncytia.

Citrus nematode (Tylenchulus semipenetrans)

Citrus nematode is a sedentary semi-endoparasite of the *Citrus* root. Females are most commonly found on thick and stunted rootlets to which a layer of soil particle is clinging. These particles are held in place by a gelatinous mucous secreted by the female. The mucous and adhering soil particles protect the females and eggs deposited by them from their natural enemies. The egg laying young females can be seen in groups clinging to rootlets with their head and neck buried in the root cortex, whereas the posterior body region found outside the root surface.

Juvenile hatches from egg in 12-14 days. Mature males develop within a week after three moults and one moult having occurred within the egg. The long slender individuals fail to develop unless they feed on a root. The second stage female juvenile requires about 14 days to locate the host root and feed on epidermal cells until ready for moulting. Fourth stage and young females are seen in about 21 days after the entry into roots. At maturity the females excrete the gelatinous matrix in which eggs are deposited. Egg laying occurs in about 40 days (Fig. 11A). The complete life cycle from egg to egg requires six to eight weeks at 25°C and reproduction occurs without the help of males.

The feeding site developed by this nematode is termed as **nurse cell,** which consists of uninucleate but not enlarged discrete parenchyma cells which are located in the cortex. Syncytium is not formed. This type of nurse cells system is characteristic for this nematode. Feeding of the citrus nematode in cortical cells results in necrosis. The injury does not extend to the stellar region of the root.

The population of the citrus nematode is closely related to the stage of decline of the trees. The nematode infestation is severe in sandy loam soil.

Reniform nematode (Rotylenchulus reniformis)

The adult female is an obligate, sedentary, semi-endoparasite of roots while the males are non-parasitic. The species is bisexual and reproduction is by amphimixis.

The species has an unusual life cycle. Although newly hatched second stage juveniles have well developed stylet, they do not feed. They soon pass through three super imposed moults to become young females and adult males. The young females force their way through cells of this tissues (Fig. 11B). During the process they feed on cortical cells. Three days after feeding, a slight swelling of the posterior body is seen and eight days, later eggs are deposited in a gelatinous matrix outside the root tissue. When these eggs are placed in water they promptly begin to hatch. The life cycle is completed in about 25 days provided the young females have found the host immediately. The nematode as a semi-endoparasite of sedentary nature, induces a specialised nurse cell systems for continuous food supply. The system involves wall expansion of several cells at the feeding site, partial wall dissolution, fusion of neighbouring cell protoplasts and finally establishment of a multinucleate syncytium. These syncytia are mostly confined to the pericycle. Other pericycle cells are metabolically stimulated but they remain discrete and uninucleate.

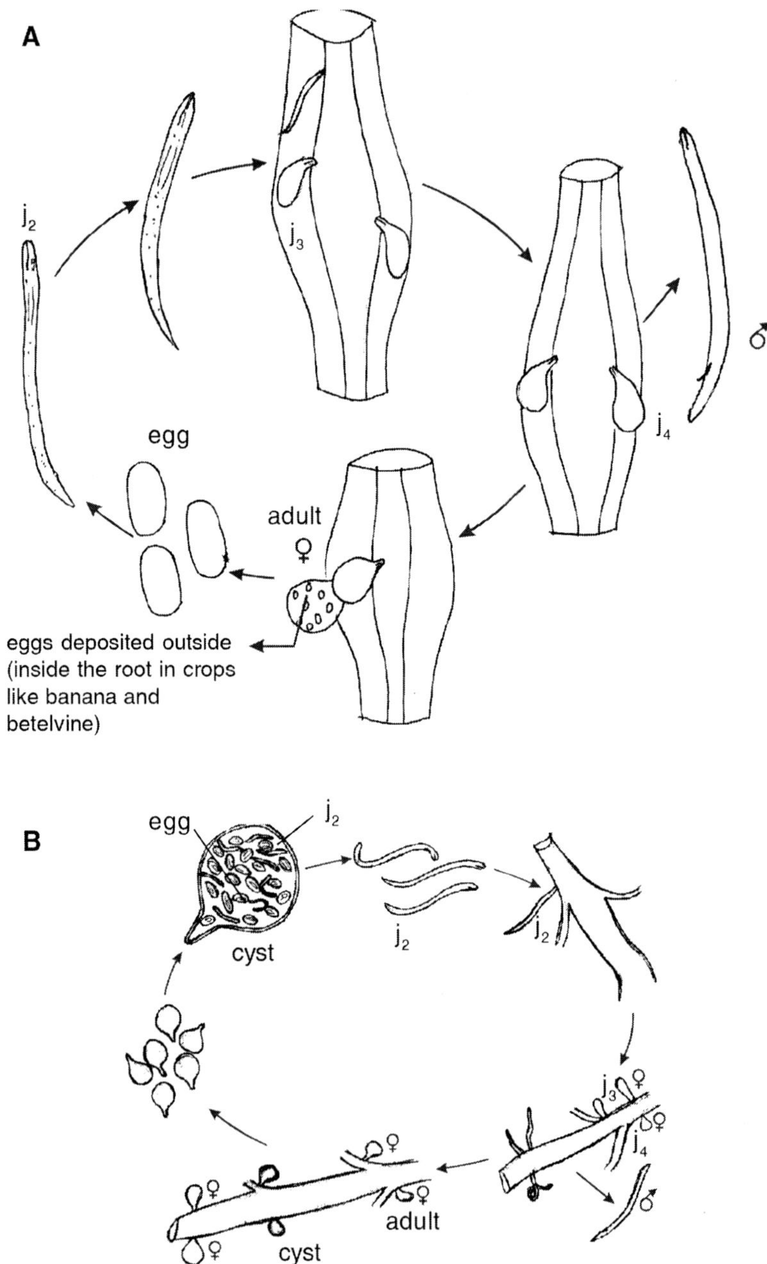

Fig. 10A: Life cycle of root-knot nematode B - Life cysle of *Globodera* spp.

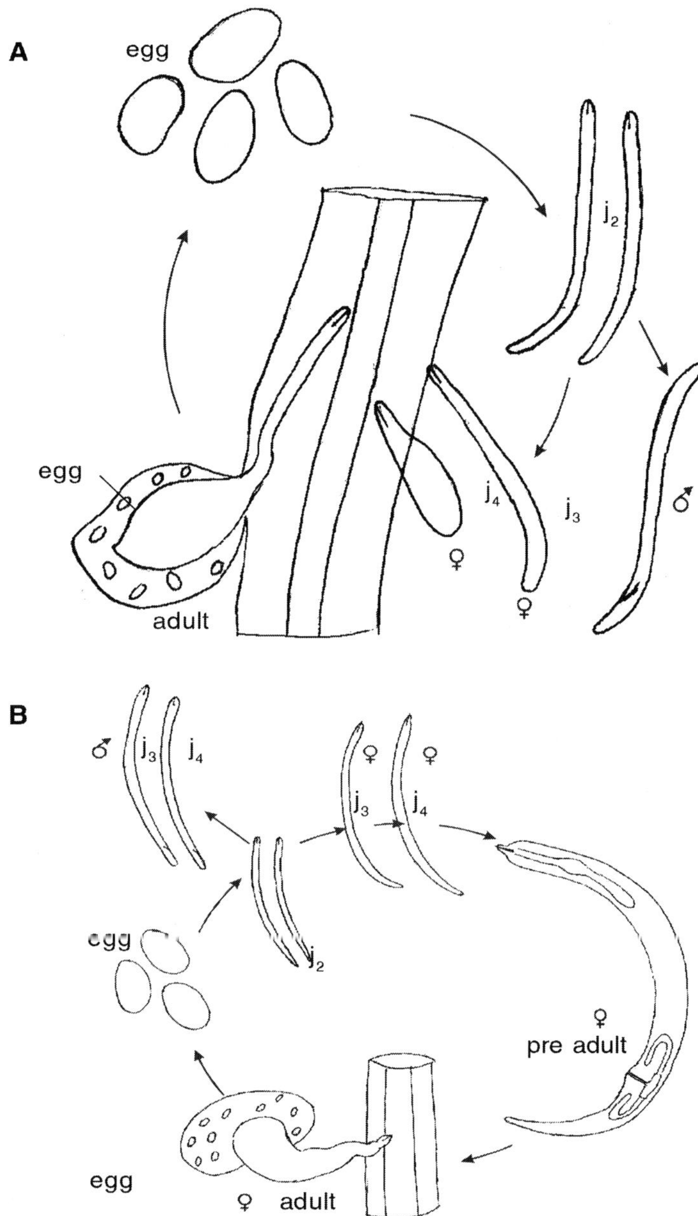

Fig. 11A: Life cycle of citrus nematode B. Life cycle of reniform nematode

The young infective females destroy the exterior cortical cells of roots and the damage increase when the nematode move towards the phloem.

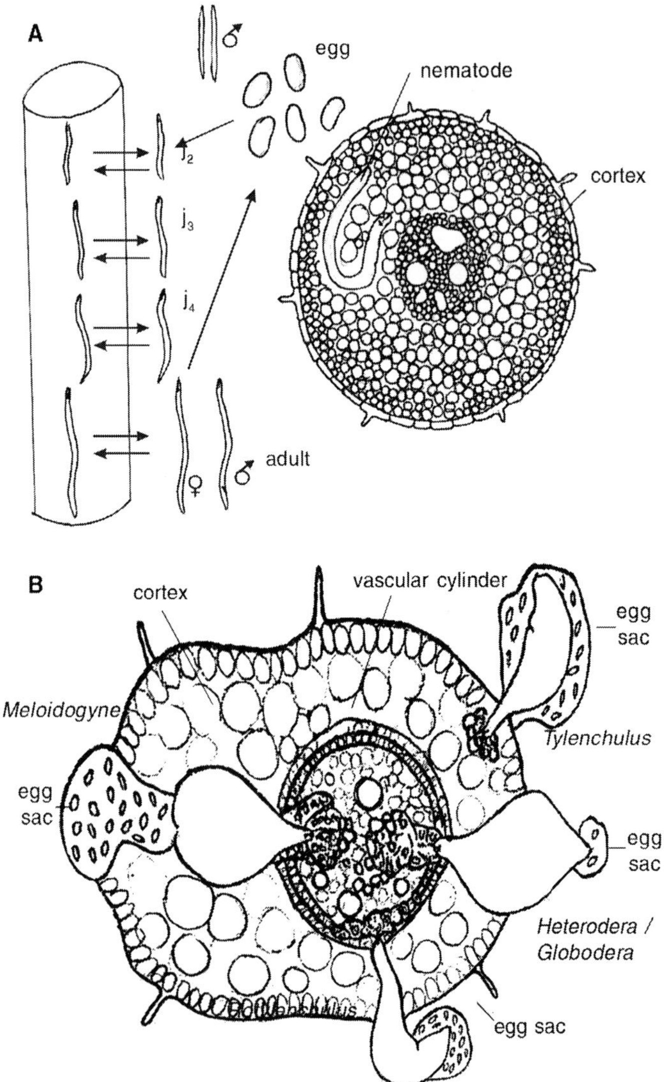

Fig. 12A: Life cycle of burrowing nematode B. Schematic representation of nurse cell systems (cross section through a root).

Burrowing nematode (Radopholus similis)

Females and all juvenile stages are infective. Males are non-parasitic and morphologically degenerate (without stylet). Penetration occurs mostly near the root tip. The nematode penetrates within 24 hours and the cells around the site of penetration becomes brown. After entering the roots, the nematodes occupy intercellular position in the cortical parenchyma where they feed on the cytoplasm of nearby cells causing cavities which coalesce to form tunnels. Nematodes do not enter the stelar portions of the root. The nematode completes its life cycle within 24-30 days at a temperature range of 21-32°C. Females lay eggs within infested tissues with an average of 4-5 eggs for two weeks (Fig. 12A). Eggs hatch after 8-10 days and the juvenile stages are completed in 10 -13 days. A low soil temperature, adequate soil moisture and availability of fresh tender roots help in the build up of population.

5

Taxonomy of Plant Parasitic Nematodes

Plant parasitic nematodes cause serious problems in sustained crop production. For a successful management of nematodes, their morphology, biology and host - parasitic relationship should be thoroughly studied. A thorough study is achieved only when its taxonomical position is known. Thus, in a simple way taxonomy can be defined as the theroretical study of classification of an organism.

The systematic arrangement of organisms into groups on the basis of their relationship is termed as classification.

Nematodes are placed in the group invertebrate, Kingdom Animalia.

Hyman (1951) revised the phylum Aschelminthes and included six classes *viz.*, Rotifera, Gastotricha, Echinodera, Priapulida, Nematoda and Nematomorpha.

Rotifera : Minute aquatic animals possessing aciliate organ. The corona located at the anterior end is provided with jaws.

Gastotricha : Similar to rotifers but lacking corona. Spines and scales are present on the body. Adhesive tubes are also present.

Echinodera : Microscopic, lacking cilia but having a segmented body with 13 – 14 segments.

Priapulida : Large marine organisms, cylindrical in shape with a superificially segmented trunk.

Nematoda : Cylindrical, vermiform, lacking cilia and presence of nerve ring posterior to mouth opening.

Nematomorpha : Filiform, similar to nematodes but without excretory system.

However, Cobb (1919) placed the nematodes under separate phylum, **Nemata / Nematoda**, which consists of two classes, Secernentea and Adenophorea.

Classification of Phylum Nematoda

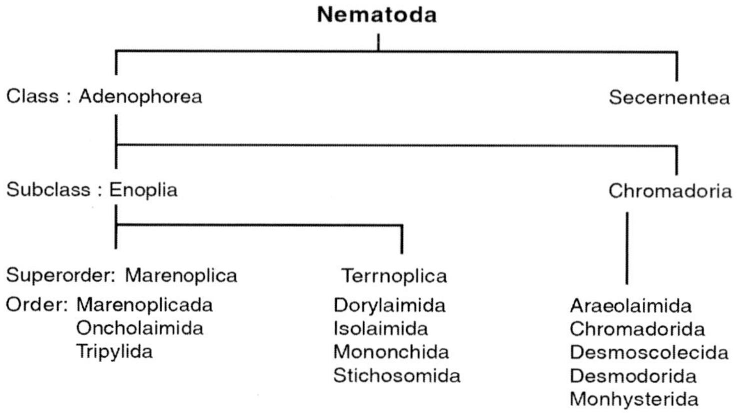

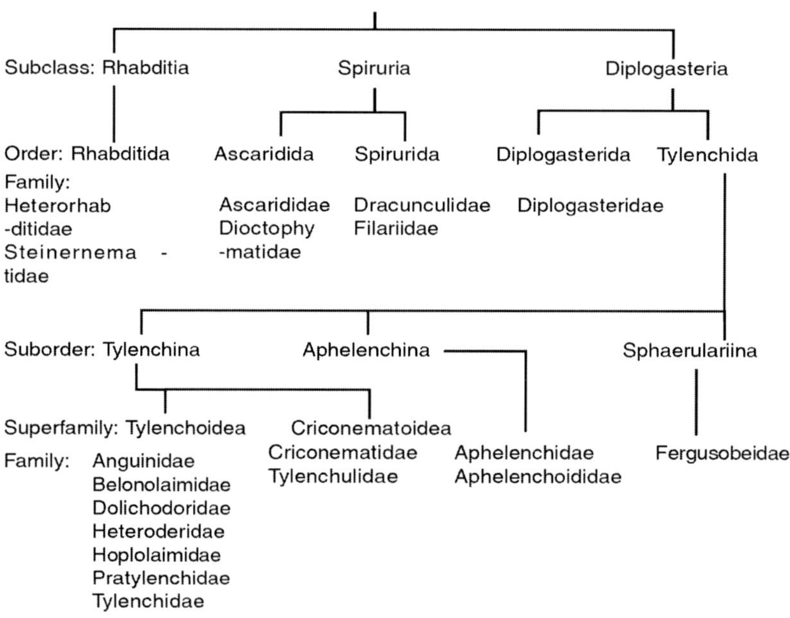

Characteristics of the phylum Nemata / Nematoda

1. The nematode possess elongate, unsegmented, cylindrical or worm like body tapering towards both ends, unciliated and circular in cross section.
2. Body is bilaterally symmertrical

3. They are aquatic, terrestrial and parasitic or free living
4. The body is covered by tough and resistant cuticle secreted by epidermal (hypodermal) cells.
5. Terminal oral aperture surrounded with lips and papillae.
6. Digestive system consists of feeding apparatus, oesophagus, intestine and rectum.
7. Body consists of two tubes.
8. The nervous system consists of nerve ring and longitudinal nerves.
9. Primitive excretory system, is devoid of protonephridial cilia or metanephiridial funnel.
10. The circulatory and respiratory systems are completely absent.
11. The females have a separate genital pore and the males have a common opening known as cloaca and well developed copulatory apparatus consisting of spicules and gubernaculum.
12. Females are oviparous or ovoviviparous or viviparous. The cleavage is terminal and growth is accompanied by moulting.
13. Life cycle is direct and there are four juvenile stages.

The plant parasitic nematodes are included in the orders Tylenchida of class Secernentea and Dorylaimida of class Adenophorea.

Secernentea (Phasmide)	Adenophorea (Aphasmida)
Arrphidial opening is on the head near the lip region	Arrphids open behind the head i.e. post labial
Laternal canals open into the excretory duct.	Lateral canals and excretory duct end in a cell
Oesophagus is divided into procorpus, median bulb, isthmus and basal bulb.	Oesophagus is cylindrical with an enlarged glandular base.
Male tail with bursa (Caudal alae)	Male tail lacks bursa but posses genital papillae.
Caudal glands are absent	Caudal glands are present
Phasmids are present	Phasmids are absent
The mesenterial tissues are less developed	The mesenterial tissues are well developed

Order: Tylenchida

Stoma armed with a protrusible spear or stomatostylet. Oesophagus consists of a procorpus, median bulb with a sclerotized valvular apparatus, nerve ring encloses the narrow isthmus and with a basal bulb. It consists of superfamilies namely Tylenchoidea, Criconematoidea, Hoplolaimoidea and Heteroderoidea.

Character	Tylenchoidea	Cri conematoidea
Labial region	Ups are hexaradiate, Labial frame work present	Labial region is poorly developed, labial plate present
Stylet	Conus, shaft and knobs are variable in shape and size	Long and anchor shaped knobs which lies in base of metacarpus
Oesophagus	Narrcw procarpus, metacarpus with valve, isthmus followed by glandular basal bulb	Pro and metacarpus amalgamated to a single unit, short isthmus, the post carpus reduced, appears as 'set off metacarpus
Dei rids	Present	Absent
Female gonad	Single or two ovary; post uterine sac (PUS) is present	Single ovary with posterior vulva; PUS absent
Male gonad	Single testis, caudal alae is present	Single testis; caudal alae rare
Phasmid	Eratically present in tail region	Not known

* The key characters of the families in the superfamily Tylenchoidea are furnished in page number ninety eight.

Differences between Tylenchina and Aphelenchina

Character	Tylenchina	Aphelenchina
Up	Varying in shape	Set - off
Annules	Faint to strong annules	Faint annules
Stylet	Well developed; one dorsal and two subventral knobs	V\feakly developed ; no stylet knobs
Oesophagus	Three parted	Three parted with square shaped median bulb
Gland bulb	Abutting, dorsal, ventral or dorsoventral overlapping on intestine	Only dorsal overlapping
Gland opening	Behind the stylet knob in procorpus	Opens in the median bulb
Female	One or two ovary; vulval position vary	Single ovary; vulva posterior
Male	Bursa present	Bursa rare
Spicule	V\feak to strong sderotization is seen with gubernaculums	Rose thorne shape spicule present

Taxonomical status and description of important plant parasitic nematodes of Tylenchoidea

Family : Dolichodoridae

Genus : *Dolichodorus* : stylet 60µ, female tail rounded to conically pointed

Family : Tylenchidae

Genus : *Tylenchus* : Female tail curved or hooked ventrally, bursa present

Family : Anguinidae

Genus : *Ditylenchus* : Thin body cuticle, stylet small with basal knobs, oesophageal gland with distinct basal bulb with a small lobe projecting part of intestine, female tail elongate and conoid, ovary one.

Genus : *Anguina* : Body cuticle thin, stylet small with basal knobs, ovary with one or two flexures, oocytes in multiple rows arranged in rachis. Occurring in wheat seed gall.

Family : Belonolaimidae

Subfamily : Tylenchorhynchinae

Genus : *Tylenchorhynchus* : Cephalic framework present, cuticle strongly annulated, ovaries two, median vulva. Stylet well developed, bursa terminal enveloping tail.

Subfamily : Belonolaiminae

Genus : *Belonolaimus* : Prominent head, deeply set off with labial disc. One incisure in lateral field, hemizonid anterior to excretory pore

Family : Pratylenchidae

Subfamily : Pratylenchinae

Genus : *Pratylenchus* : Oesophageal gland overlaps the intestine ventrally, single ovary.

Subfamily : Radopholinae

Genus : *Radopholus* : Oesophageal gland overlaps the intestine dorsally, tail terminus rounded. Two ovaries.

Genus : *Hirschmanniella* : Large nematode, tail terminus pointed with mucron.

Family : Nacobbidae

Genus : *Nacobbus* : Dorsal oesophageal gland opens close to the base of stylet, single ovary, bursa enveloping tail.

Family : Hoplolaimidae

Subfamily : Hoplolaiminae

Genus : *Hoplolaimus* : Well developed cephalic frame work, phasmids large not opposite to each other, stylet well developed, massive basal knobs with anterior projections, two ovaries.

Genus : *Scutellonema* : Large phasmids opposite to each other on tail

Genus : *Helicotylenchus* : Dorsal oesophageal gland open away from the base of stylet, ventral overlapping

Subfamily : *Rotylenchus* : Dorsal oesophageal gland open near the base of stylet, dorsal overlapping of oesophageal gland, two ovaries, males with weak stylet, adanal bursa.

Family : Heteroderidae

Subfamily : Heteroderinae

Genus : *Heterodera* : pyriform or lemon shape; female body becoming cyst

Genus : *Globodera* : round or globular cysts

Subfamily : Meloidogyninae

Genus : *Meloidogyne* : body cuticle thin, without spines, vulva and anus close together and terminal, eggs laid in gelatinous matrix. Adult female pyriform with tapering neck.

Family : Aphelenchoididae

Subfamily : Aphelenchoidinae

Genus : *Aphelenchoides* : Body less slender, tail short, conical, male without bursal flap

Subfamily : Rhadinaphelenchinae

Genus : *Rhadinaphelenchus* : body extremely slender; terminal bursal flap present

Subfamily : Bursaphelenchinae

Genus : *Bursaphelenchus* : Head set off, spear weak, thorne shape spicule, bursa at tail tip.

Family : Criconematidae

Subfamily : Criconematinae

Genus : *Criconema* : Annules coarse with cuticular spines or scale like projections extending posteriorly

Genus : *Hemicriconemoides* : Adult female with prominent cuticular sheath

Subfamily : Hemicycliophorinae

Genus : *Hemicycliophora* : Female more elongate, stylet knobs spherical, sloping posteriorly. Adult female with cuticular sheath

Family : Tylenchulidae

Subfamily : Tylenchulinae

Genus : *Tylenchulus* : Excretory pore sub - equatorial and anterior to vulva

Subfamily : Paratylenchinae

Genus : *Paratylenchus* : female slender with short tail

Superfamily Criconematoidea

Family

Criconematidae	Tylenchulidae
Cuticle heavily annulated with spines and scale like projections extending posteriorly, cuticlular sheath present	Finely annulated, stylet well developed, female sub spherical and saccate.
Subfamilies: Criconematinae Hemicycliophorinae	Tylenchulinae Paratylenchinae

Order : Dorylaimid

The labial region is set off from body contour. The stoma is armed with a movable mural tooth or a hollow axial spear. Oesophagus is divided into a slender, muscular anterior region and an elongated or pyriform glandular posterior region. Females have one or two reflected ovaries, males have paired equal spicules, gubernaculums rare. The order is divided into three sub orders namely Dorylaimina, Diphtherophodrina and Nygolaimina. The former two suborders containing the plant parasitic nematodes.

Sub order

Dorylaimina	Diptherophodrina
Stylet with flanges or guiding	Teeth like spear, solid, short ring, long and straight and ventrally curved
Family : Longidoridae	Trichodoridae

Family : Longidoridae

Genus : *Longidorus* : amphids pouch like, slit like opening, spear extension without flanges, guiding ring located near the spear tip

Genus : *Xiphinema* : amphids funnel shaped wide opening, spear extension with flanges, guiding ring located near the spear base.

Family : Trichodoridae

Genus : *Trichodorus* : Long curved onchiostylet, female rectum runs parallel to the longitudinal body axis and the anus lies subterminally. Male tail curved, bursa absent, vaginal sclerotization strong, lateral pores present near vulva.

The key identification characters and diagrams are furnished for important plant parasitic nematodes.

Stunt Nematode (*Tylenchorhynchus*)

Parasitism and habitat

Ectoparasitic on many plants and rarely endoparasitic. All stages are found in the rhizosphere.

Main morphological characters

Body	: 0.6 - 1.4 mm in length
Lip	: Typically continuous with body or slightly set off
Stylet	: Usually strong with large basal knobs
Oesophagus	: Typically with procorpus, metacorpus and well developed posterior bulb without over lapping the intestine
Ovaries	: Two
Vulva	: Almost near the middle of the body

Tail : In female it is tapering to rounded, usually one or more times as long as anal body diameter

Resembling genera : *Tylenchus* (In this genera only one ovary is present and vuvla located in the posterior region) and *Psilenchus* (the tail is slender and longer)

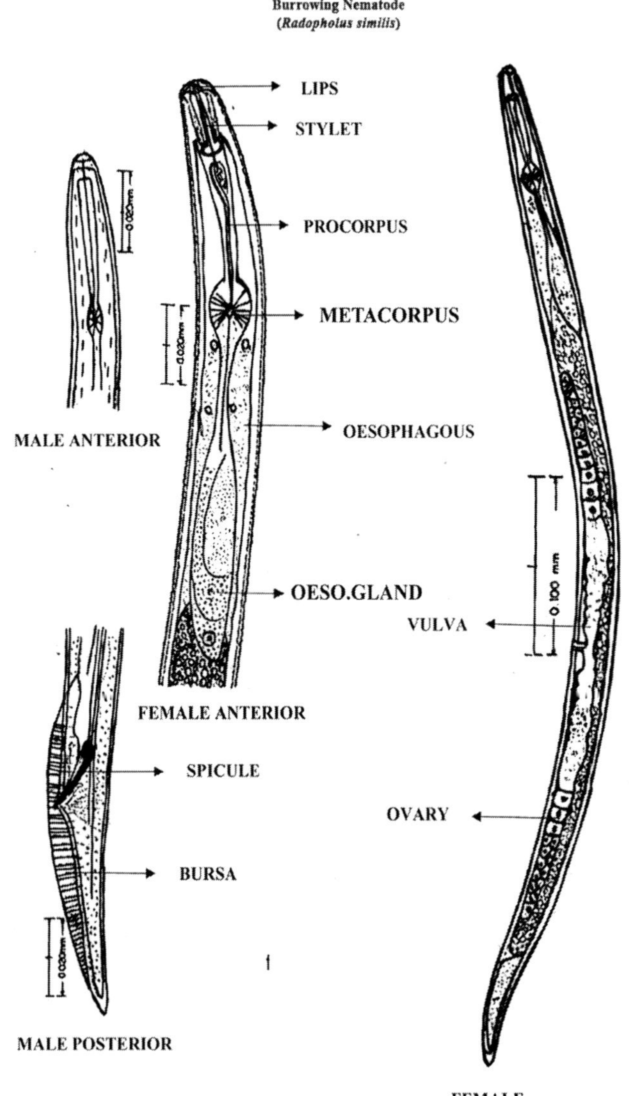

Burrowing nematode (*Radopholus*)

Parasitism and habitat

Endoparasitic on few plants particularly on banana and citrus. All stages are found in root tissues and in the rhizosphere.

Main morphological characters

Body : 0.4 - 0.9 mm

Lip : Typically round in female and in males set off and knob like.

Stylet : Short and stout in female and it is very slender and rudimentary.

Oesophagus : Forming a lobe, dorsally overlap the intestine.

Ovaries : Two

Vulva : Located at the middle of the body

Tail : Tapers to a blunt end in female and in male the tail is long with bursa.

Resembling genus : *Hirschmanniella* (This genus is slender and long compared to *R. similis*).

Lance Nematode (*Hoplolaimus*)

Parasitism and habitat

Ectoparasitic and endoparasitic on many plants. All stages are found in soil or root.

Main morphological characters

Body : Length of males and females ranges from 1.0 to 2.0 mm

Lip : Typically set-off with annules divided into small segments (visible under oil immersion).

Stylet : Strongly developed with typically elongated and closely arranged basal knobs

Oesophagus : With median bulb; Oesophageal glands with short lobe overlapping dorsally to the anterior end of intestine

Ovaries : Two

Vulva : Centrally located

Bursa : Present

Resembling genus : *Scutellonema* and *Rotylenchus* (Stylet knobs broader and male tail shorter in these two genera)

Helicotylenchus (Dorsal gland orifice located at least one half of the stylet length posterior to stylet)

Spiral nematode (*Helicotylenchus*)

Parasitism and habitat

Endoparasitic and ectoparasitic on many plants; all stages are found in soil and root.

Main morphological characters

Body : Typically arcuate or spiral in shape when dead or relaxed. Length from 0.5 to 1.2 mm

Stylet : Moderately long

Dorsal oesophageal: Typically located more than one – half stylet gland orifice length posterior to stylet knobs

Ovaries : Two

Vulva : Posterior to middle of body (60 – 70%)

Tail : In females, round to nearly pointed; often with short projection on ventral side and in males the tail is short with bursa

Resembling genus : *Hoplolaimus*, *Scutellonema* and *Rotylenchus*

Lesion nematode (*Pratylenchus*)

Parasitism and habitat

Migratory endoparasite, feeding in root cortex of many plants. All stages are found in root or soil. Males common in many species, unknown or less common in others.

Main morphological characters

Body length : 0.4 - 0.8 mm

Lip region : Slightly set-off from body

Stylet : Typically short, strong with massive knobs

Ovary : Typically one and posterior ovary rudimentary to form a post uterine sac

Vulva : Typically on the posterior fourth of the body (75 – 80%)

Tail : Nearly round to pointed and in the case of male, tail has bursa

Resembling genus : *Radopholus* (Two ovaries present instead of one and great morphological diffrence between male and females observed in *Radopholus*)

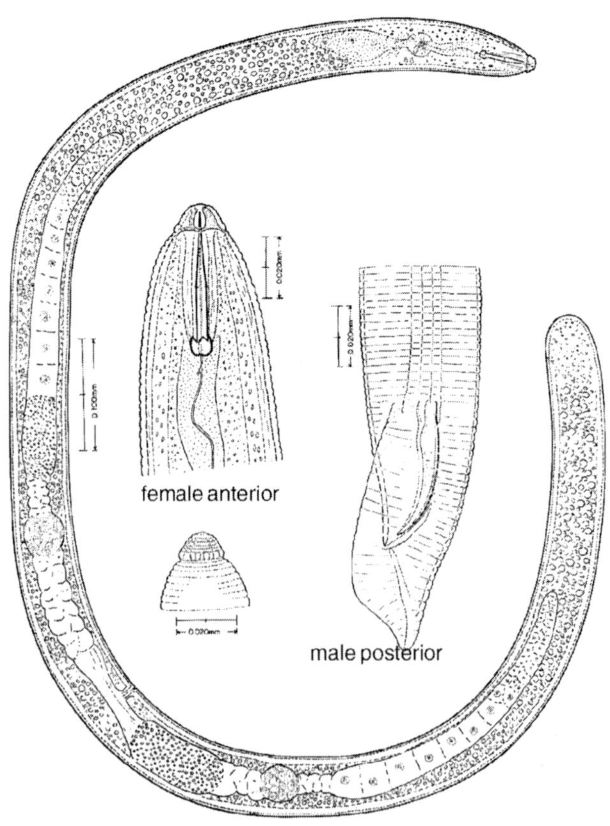

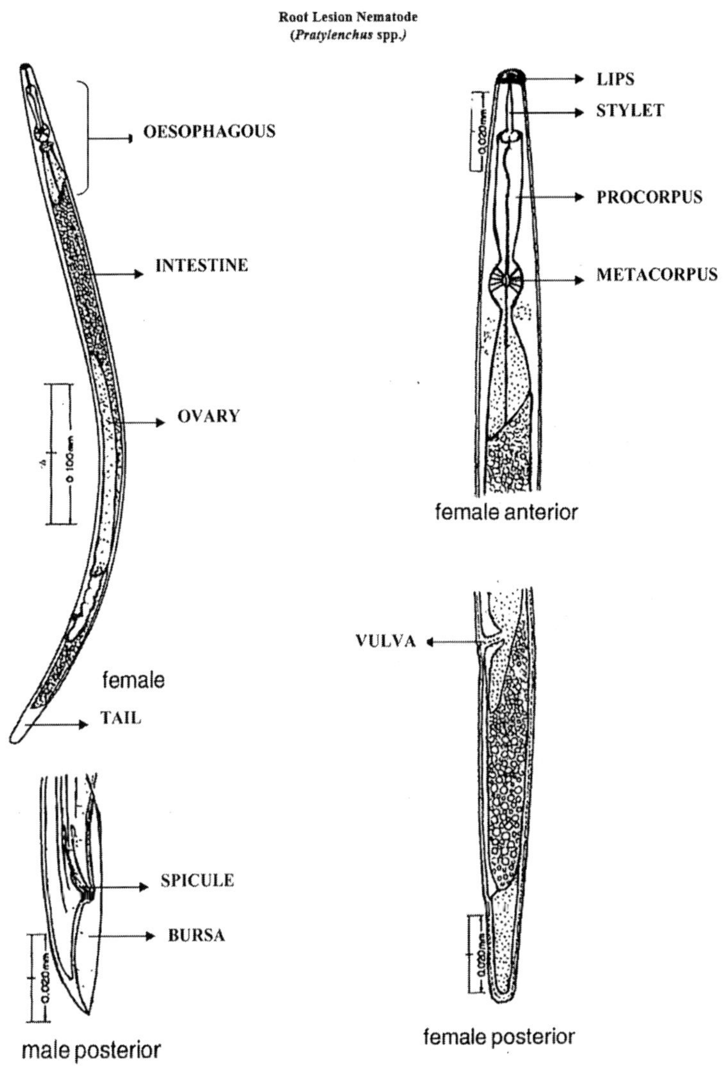

Rice-root nematode (*Hirschmanniella*)

Parasitism and habitat

Endoparasitic on rice, grasses sedges etc.

Main morphological characters

Body	: Typically long, slender (1.2 to 3.0 mm or more) and annulated
Stylet	: Typically short with rounded knobs
Vulva	: Typically near the middle of the body
Ovary	: Median, ovaries two and amphidelphic
Oesophagus	: With conspicuous median bulb; oesophageal glands in a lobe, overlapping anterior end of the intestine ventrally.
Tail	: Bluntly pointed with short sharp projections; male tail long with bursa
Resembling genus	: *Radopholus* (body much shorter, always less than 1.0 mm and sharp projection on the tail is absent)

Rice Root Nematode
(*Hirschmanniella*)

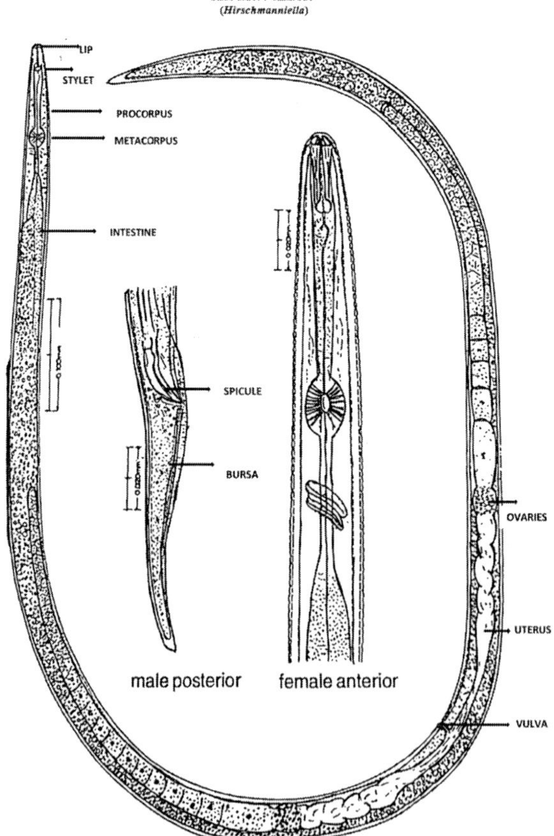

Ring nematode (*Criconemoides*)

Parasitism and habitat

Ectoparasitic on many plants; female and juveniles found in soil, males seldom or never found.

Main morphological characters

Body : Typically short (0.3 to 0.8 mm), wide with large annules in female and juveniles nearly always with angular posterior edge. Annules of males are much smaller

Stylet : Typically of medium size; often absent in males

Oesophagus : With median bulb and has narrow posterior bulb

Oesophageal lumen: Lying in coils above median bulb valve when stylet not exserted.

Ovary : Only one

Vulva : Located near the posterior part of body

Tail : Bluntly rounded to pointed in females

Resembling genus : *Criconema* (Hingly variable scales or spines present on posterior edge of annules. In some intermediate forms, adults have poorly developed spines; in others, scales are present in juveniles only)

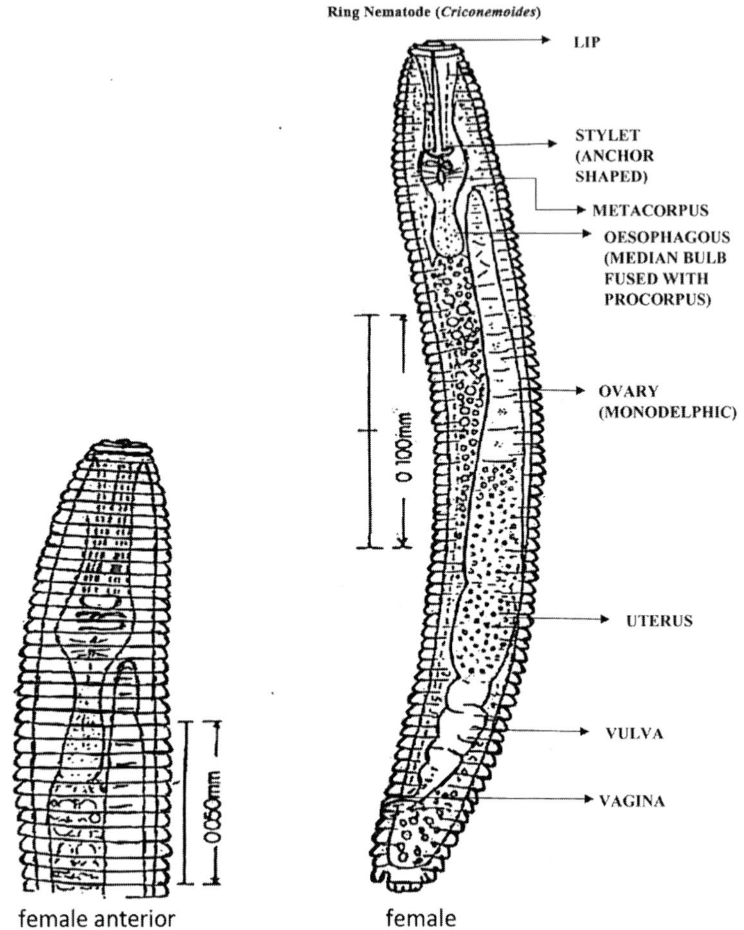

Sheath nematode (*Hemicycliophora*)

Parasitism and habitat

Ectoparasitic on various plants, sometimes associated with distinct, irregularly shaped galls on young roots. Females, males and juveniles are found. Males of many species have not been found in the soil.

Main morphological characters

Body : Length varies from 0.8 to 2.0 mm in females 0.4 to 1.0 mm in males. In females, body typically covered by a sheath looking like cuticle in the process of moulting. No

	sheath in males. Shape more or less semicircular in some species
Stylet	: Slender, elongated with well developed basal bulbs in females and stylet is absent in males
Oesophagus	: Well developed in females with median bulb, anterior end fused together and posterior bulb rather short; degenerate in males.
Ovary	: Only one present
Vulva	: Located in the posterior region of the body
Tail	: In females from pointed to bluntly rounded; in males conical to pointed.
Spicules	: Typically large and curved
Bursa	: Present
Resembling genus	: *Criconemoides*

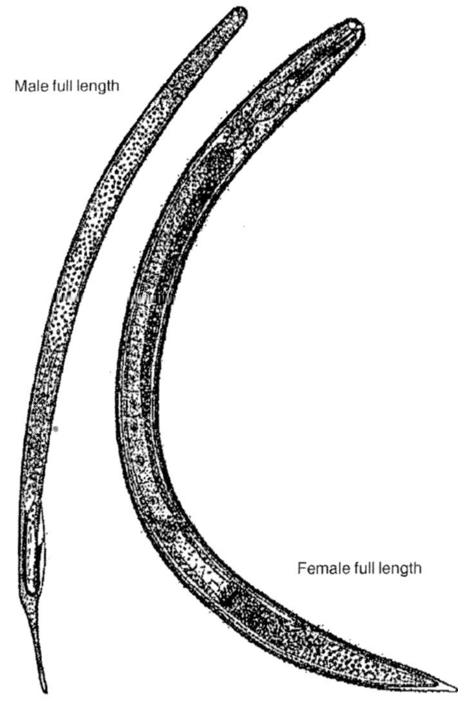

Hemciycliophora

Sting nematode (*Belonolaimus*)

Parasitism and habitat

Ectoparasitic on various plants. Males and females found in the soil.

Main morphological characters

Body : Female body long and slender (2.0 to 3.0 mm); in male the body is slightly smaller (19.5 to 2.5 mm). the lateral field is a single line extending to full length of the body

Lip region : Hemispherical

Stylet : Typically very long and slender attached to the oesophageal lumen. This lies coiled above the valve of the median oesophageal bulb when stylet is not exserted

Tail : Female tail cylindrical with rounded tip and in male the tail is very long, pointed and with bursa

Gubernaculum : Varying with species by usually with a posterior projection

Resembling genus: *Dolichodorus* (tails of females sharply pointed and of males short)

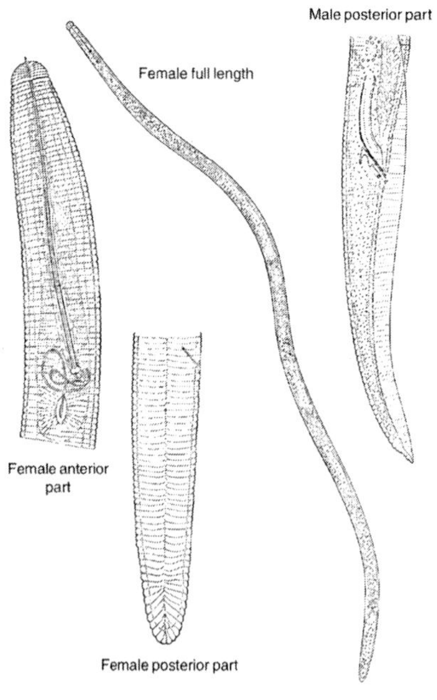

Belonolaimus

Root - knot nematode (*Meloidogyne*)

Parasitism and habitat

Females as well as third and fourth stage juvenile are sedentary endoparasites on many plants. Males and second stage juvenile are migratory and can be located in soil also.

Main morphological characters

Body	: Elongate juvenile (0.5 mm) and males (1.0 – 2.0 mm); typically saccate, spheroid with a distinct neck in females (0.8 mm long and 0.5 mm wide)
Stylet	: Strong with rounded knobs in males ; in females more slender than in males or juveniles but with strong basal knobs
Oesophagus	: With very large median bulb followed by a short isthmus
Excretory pore	: Often seen with part of excretory tube in the area between posterior part of stylet knobs and opposite to median bulb
Vulva and anus	: In females, typically opposite to neck and surrounded by a pattern of fine lines resembling human fingerprints. (These are used for identification of species in this genus)
Spicules	: Very near the terminus of males ; bursa absent
Resembling genus	: *Heterodera*

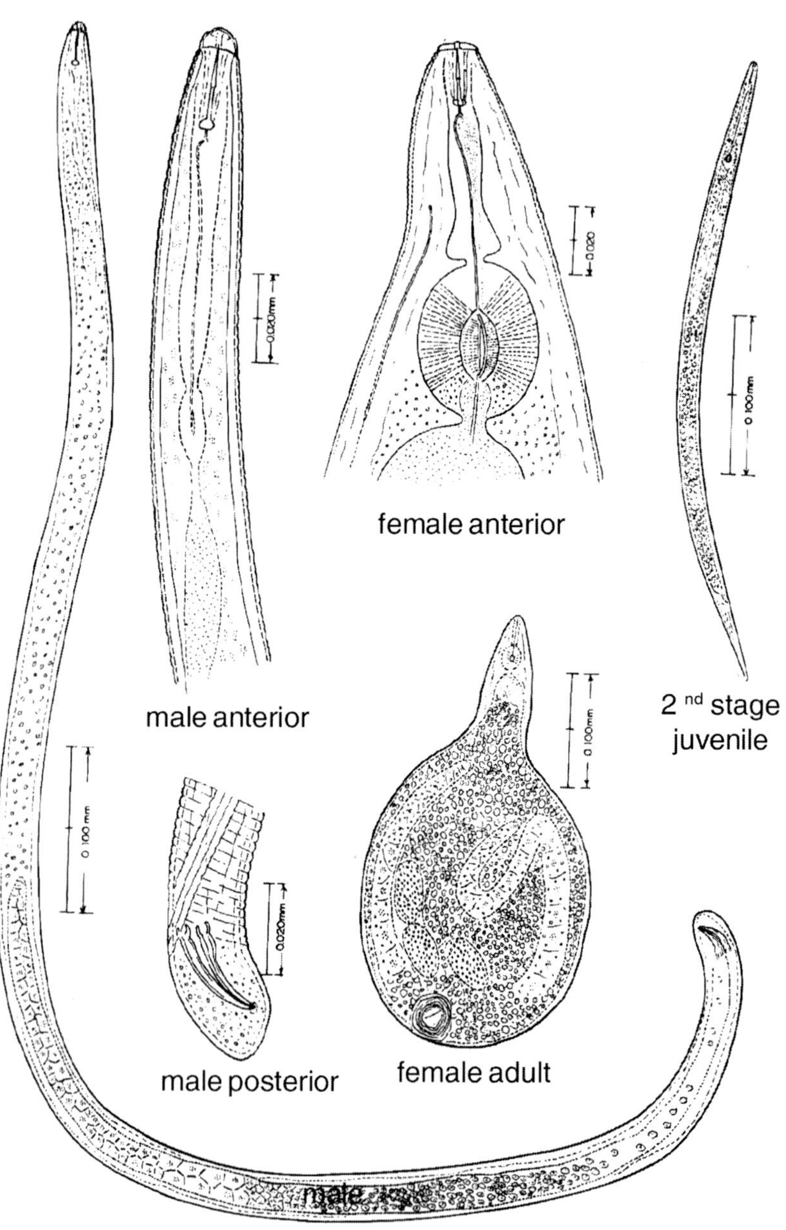

Meloidogyne

Cyst nematode (*Heterodera*)

Parasitism and habitat

Parasitic on many plants mostly in temperate zone (notably potato, sugarbeet, oat and other grains, clover, soybean and various crucifers). Adult females with neck embedded in plant roots and the body exposed. Juveniles, males and cysts found in soil.

Main morphological characters

Body : Slender in males (1.0 to 2.0 mm) and juveniles (0.3 to 0.6 mm); in females, typically swollen lemon-shaped (0.5-0.8 mm in length), white or yellow in colour. Cysts dark brown, lemon shaped (0.8mm long and 0.5mm wide) or nearly the same shape as that of *Meloidogyne* female.

Stylet : Short in males with rounded basal knobs and in juveniles, more than 0.02mm long

Oesophagus : With well developed median bulb and lobe extending back and overlapping the intestine

Spicules : Near the posterior end of females

Resembling genus : *Meloidogyne* (stylet of juveniles only 0.01-0.014 mm long; adult females fully embedded in roots in case of *Meloidogyne*)

Potato cyst nematode :(*Globodera*): The adult females are globular in shape and hence, the genus is named as *Globodera*

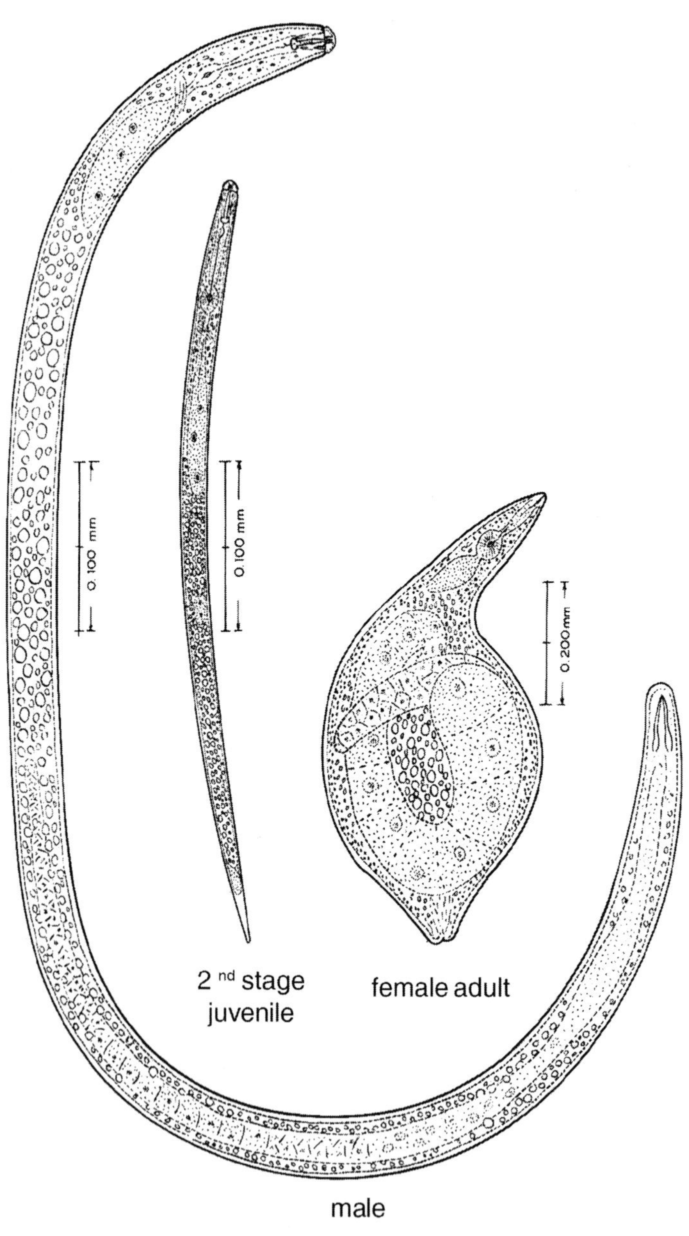

Heterodera

Citrus nematode (*Tylenchulus*)

Parasitism and habitat

Endoparasitic on roots of citrus and other plants. Slender young females, males and juveniles are found in soil (where they can be easily overlooked or mistaken for juveniles of other species). In case of mature females they protrude from roots, often in clusters as semiendoparasites.

(Note : Mature females are usually masked by egg masses to which soil particles adhere. For best observation, remove egg mass).

Main morphological characters

Body length : Small in all stages (0.20 – 0.50 mm); in mature females, typically swollen

Stylet : Small in juveniles and males and well developed in young females

Oesophagus : With distinct posterior bulb in juveniles; young males and immature females.

Vulva : Prominent in the posterior end of young and adult females

Excretory pore : Typically situated posteriorly in a protuberance just anteriror to the vulva.

Anus : Absent or difficult to see in all immature stages

Bursa : Absent

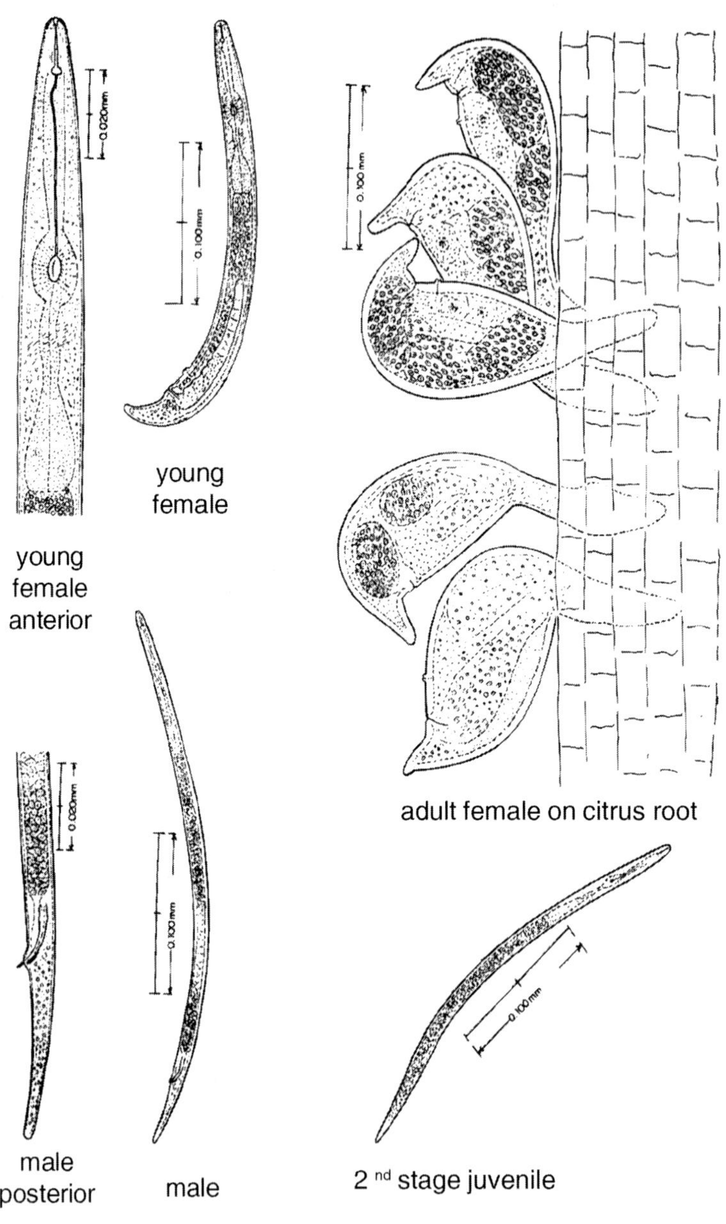

Tylenchulus

Reniform nematode (*Rotylenchulus*)

Parasitism and habitat

Parasitic on many plants. Mature females with only their neck embedded in roots as semiendoparasites (difficult to see because covered with egg masses and soil particles); juveniles, males and immature females are found in soil.

Main morphological characters

Body	: Slender and small in males (0.30 to 0.50 mm), immature females (0.30 to 0.45 mm) and juveniles (0.30 to 0.45 mm); typically reniform (kidney- shaped) in adult females (0.60 to 0.90 mm)
Oesophagus	: Dorsal oesophageal gland typically open about one stylet length posterior to stylet knobs
Resembling genus	: *Tylenchulus*

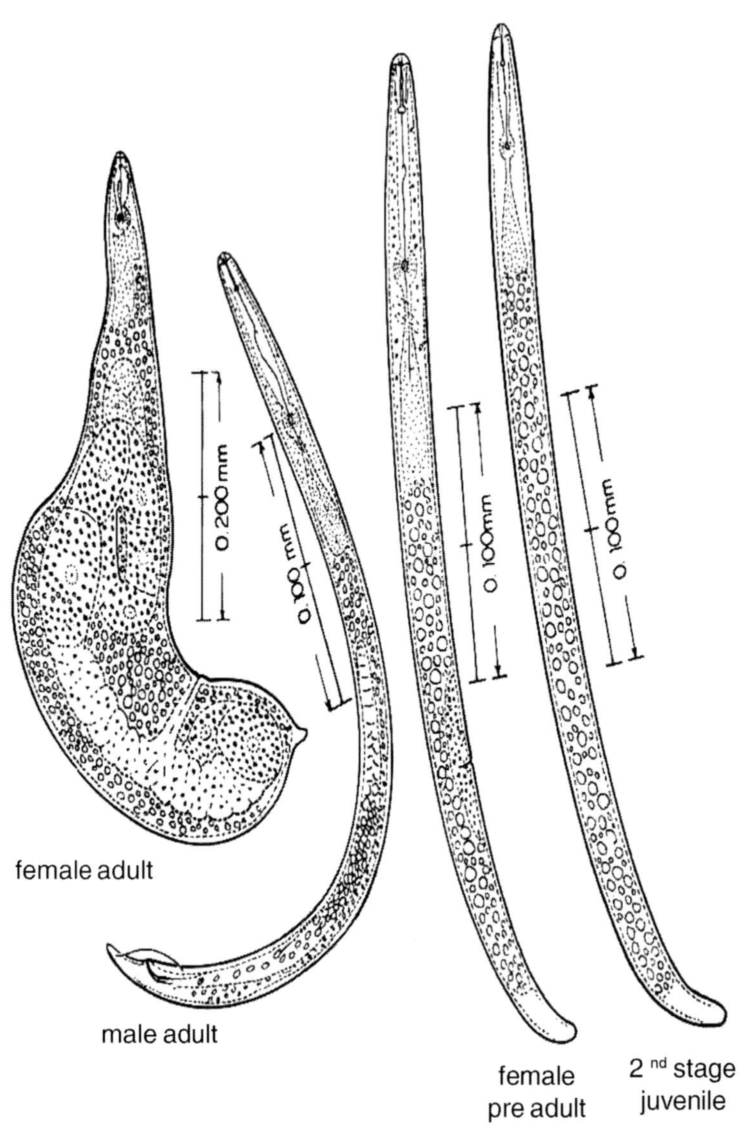

Rotylenchulus

Dagger nematode (*Xiphinema*)

Parasitism and habitat

Ectoparasitic on many plants and often associated with perennial plants. All stages are found in the rhizosphere.

Main morphological characters

Body	: Typically long (1.5 to 5.0 mm), slender without annulations
Stylet	: Typically long, very slender having flanged knobs and "guiding ring" located near the base of the stylet
Oesophagus	: Anterior tube slender and the posterior part wide
Ovaries	: One or Two
Vulva	: Located near the middle of the body or near end of oesophagus when only one ovary is present
Tail	: Bluntly rounded or with projection on the ventral side
Resembling genus	: *Longidorus* and *Paralongidorus* (in these two genera flanged stylet knobs absent and guiding ring located near anterior end of the stylet)

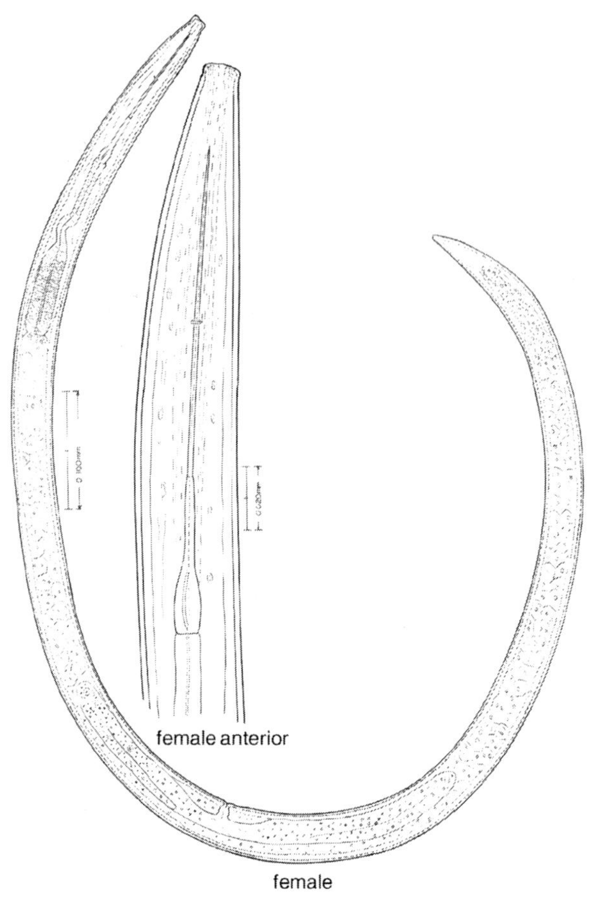

Xiphinema

Stubby – root nematode (*Trichodorus*)

arasitism and habitat

Ectoparasitic on many plants. All stages are found in soil.

Main morphological characters

Body	: 0.4 - 1.5 mm
Stylet	: Solid, typically curved dorsally, without knobs
Oesophagus	: With typical pyriform basal bulb
Ovaries	: Usually two
Vulva	: Near middle of the body
Tail	: Bluntly rounded in both female and male
Anus	: Near posterior end

Charecter	Tylenchidae	Anguluidae	Dolichodoridae	Belenolaimidae	Pratylenchidae	Hoplolamidae	Heteroderidae
Body	Sender,vermiform	Sender. Swollen wark	Long and slender	Sender, robust	Elongate, slender	vermiform to kidney shape	Male vermiform female saccate
Labia	Elevated, round, annulated	Lew, flatten	Distinctly set-off annulated	High, rounded	Lew	High, set-off round, trapezoid	Round, annulated
Labial frame wark	Yfesk	Highly scelerotized	Heavily sclerotized	Poor to well developed	Well developed	Srong and well developed	Well developed
Lateral field	1 to many lines	4,6 or more	64	2-6	2-4	4	2-4; faintly seen
Stylet	Small and delicate	Small and delicate	Long, well developed	Long	Short and stout	Srong	Well developed
Oesophagus	Narrow procarpus, elliptical metacarpus, slender isthmus pyriform basal bulb	Basal bulb pyriform irregularly shaped	Amalgamated pro & metacarpus pyriform basal bulb, no overlapping	Sender procarpus round metacarpus slim isthmus pyriform basal bulb	Three parted, ventral overlapping	Dorsal overlapping	Dorsal overlapping
Female	IVbno-prodelphic, post uterine sac present (PUS)	Mono-prodelphic, reflated	Ddelphic amphidelphic	Ddelphic amphidelphic	IVbno-prodelphic PUS present	Ddelphic amphidelphic	Ddelphic prodelphic
Male	IVbnorchic, Laptoderan bursa	Leptoderan & Reloderan	Fteloderan	Fteloderan	Ffeloderan	Fteloderan	No bursa
Tail	Elongate, conoid, pyriform or variable in shape	Conoid	Blunty rounded	Cylinderical to conoid	Trapezoidal, variable	Blunty rounded	Conoid to pointed

6

Nematological Techniques

Sampling for nematode population estimation

Sampling for nematode communities has been the basis for the development of appropriate control strategy. The major purposes of sampling for nematodes include population estimation for general detection, advisory or predictive programme, disease diagnosis and also for research purposes.

Plant parasitic nematodes are usually confined to top 20-25 cm soil and may vary depending upon the soil type, moisture content, host plant and climatic condition. Surface soil do not harbour any nematode. The roots and rhizosphere of severely infested plants do not harbour numerous nematodes as the nematodes tend to move to adjacent healthy plants. Hence soil and root samples need to be collected from plants showing partial symptoms. Samples should not be collected from dead or wilted plants.

B. Collection of soil and root samples for nematode extraction:

Materials required	:	Trowel, shovel, soil auger, soil core probe or hand hoe, polythene bag, label, rubber band, pencil and knife

Sampling for Nematode population estimation in different cropping systems

1. Sampling from field crops

- Leave about 1 m peripheral area of the field.
- Remove 2-3 cm upper layer of the soil with the help of a hand hoe.
- Collect 200 cc soil along with feeder roots up to a depth of 15-20 cm (subsample). Draw 10-20 such subsamples from one hectare area in a zig zag manner.
- Put all the subsamples in the same polythene bag (composite sample).
- Reduce the composite sample by quartering method to have a representative sample.

- Put an aluminium foil label or paper bearing the sample number and other details in the polythene bag and tie it with a rubber band.

2. Sampling from vegetable crops

- Select 6 rows of a field (2 from the beginning, 2 from the middle and 2 from the far end of the field).
- Collect 8-10 subsamples up to a depth of 20-30 cm from each pair of rows in a zig zag manner.
- Put all the subsamples in the same polythene bag and label it.
- Reduce the composite sample by quartering method (representative sample).

3. Sampling from an orchard

- Take two subsamples from one tree up to a depth of 30 to 60 cm (feeder root zone) depending upon the age of the tree.
- Collect subsamples from 10 trees randomly from one hectare area.
- Pool all the subsamples in the same polythene bag and label it.
- Reduce the composite sample by quartering method (representative sample).

Sampling from a tree

- Collect 5 subsamples each from around the main stem and drip line of the tree by the method described above.
- The depth of the sampling will vary with the kind and age of the tree.
- Put all the subsamples in the same polythene bag and label it.
- Reduce the composite sample by quartering method (representative sample).

Labeling

Write sample number and details on an aluminium foil or paper label, fold it and put in the polythene bag. Tie the mouth of the polythene bag with a rubber band. Label should contain the following information.

- Location and sample number
- Host/crop and stage of crop

- Variety
- Previous crop
- Condition of the crop
- Date of sampling
- Soil type
- Name of the sample collector
- Farmer's name and address

Important precautions

- Select live plants showing symptoms.
- Take samples from the rhizosphere.
- Avoid sampling immediately after fertilizer or pesticide application and irrigation or heavy rainfall.
- Avoid surface soil pebbles and plant debris.
- Keep the plant materials moist in polythene bags.

Care and storage of samples

Plant parasitic nematodes are thin walled, short lived microorganisms. Improper handling such as exposure to the sun, temperature extremes of improper storage results in high mortality rates. The handling of soil and root samples during collection and transit to the laboratory warrant special care. After collection, each sample should be sealed in a plastic bag and placed in an insulated container or kept out of the sun at a moderate temperature, preferably less than 30 °C. Exposure to the sun or high temperature leads to death of the nematodes.

Storage

Temperature and soil moisture are the critical parameters that affect nematode survival in storage. It is recommended to store the samples at 10-15 °C. Normally the samples can be stored in BOD incubator setting a temperature between 10-15 °C or in a refrigerator at 4 °C.

Extraction of nematodes from soil / Cobb's decanting and sieving method (Cobb, 1918)

This method is based on the principle of gravity. Here, the difference in size and specific gravity between nematodes and other soil components are utilized. Heavier particles settle down more easily compared to the lighter ones. Nematodes being lighter in weight can be separated out from other matter using the principle of gravity.

A set of sieves with specific mesh number is used for this purpose. The mesh numbers and pore aperture are as follows.

Mesh number	Pore aperture (m)
20	840
60	250
100	150
200	75
350	45

Collection of sample

A detailed sampling plan, such as the sampling pattern, number and size of cores per sample have to be assessed. The number of samples is need to be worked out based on theoretical and practical consideration.

Sampling equipment

Equipment for collecting soil samples for nematode assays includes, hand trowel or garden shovel, soil augers or tubes. The typical cylindrical tube type sampler or auger is used as a standard equipment by many nematologists. The tubes of 20-25 mm diameter are used frequently. Fifty cores from these tubes give about 2 kg of soil. Apart from this, polythene bag, label and rubber bands are also required to collect and secure the samples.

Timing of sample

Timing of sample collection is depending on the purpose of the nematode assay and the population dynamics of the target species. Survey samples for use in quarantines or in the characterization of nematode distribution should be made when nematode population occur in maximum numbers. For evaluation of nematicide three to four sample period should be employed. For nematicide treatments, a pre-treatment sample within one week prior to treatment, an intermediate post-treatment, a midseason and a final sample should be taken. Weekly or biweekly nematode and plant monitoring may be neccessary in modelling experiments.

Sample size

Sample size may be determined on the basis of relative population densities and the nematode spatial pattern. Ten sampling units may provide an adequate estimates of a large population. For low population densities 100 sampling units are neccessary.

Sampling pattern

Sampling patterns used for nematode assay include random, stratified random, systematic and two stage sampling. The specific type or spatial pattern and relative density of the target nematode species should be considered in selection of the sampling procedure.

The step-by-step procedure is as follows (Fig. 13)

1. Mix the soil sample thoroughly and place 250 ml of the sample using a 250 ml plastic beaker into a 5 litre plastic bucket or basin A.
2. Add 2 litres of water to the plastic bucket and mix thoroughly.
3. Hold the bucket for about 10 seconds to permit the heavy soil particles and stones to settle down. Then decant by passing through a coarse sieve (mesh number 20) into another plastic bucket B. During this process the nematodes are carried to the plastic bucket B along with the water suspension. The plant debris and stones are collected in the 20 mesh sieve which can be discarded.
4. The contents of the bucket B are mixed again and hold it for 10 seconds and decant the suspension through a fine sieve (350 mesh) where the nematodes will be retained in the sieve. (Use 200 mesh sieve before using 350 mesh sieve if the soil is more of humus, silt and clay). Repeat the process once again using the same 350 mesh to ensure cent per cent collection of the nematode in the fine sieve.
5. The contents of 350 mesh sieve may be washed using a squeeze bottle with a slow jet of water to remove soil as far as possible and transfer the nematode suspension into a plastic beaker.

   Modified Baermann's Funnel Method

6. Pour the nematode suspension into a wire gauze containing a layer of tissue paper kept in a Petri dish (Modified Baermann's funnel) holding sufficient water to be in contact with the bottom of the wire gauze.
7. Leave the Funnel or Petri dish overnight (12h). During this period of time, the nematodes move by penetrating through the minute pores in

the tissue paper and settle in the water (Fig. 14). Collect the nematode suspension in the funnel or Petri dish for counting. The nematodes can be counted with the aid of a counting dish by taking 5 ml of nematode suspension.

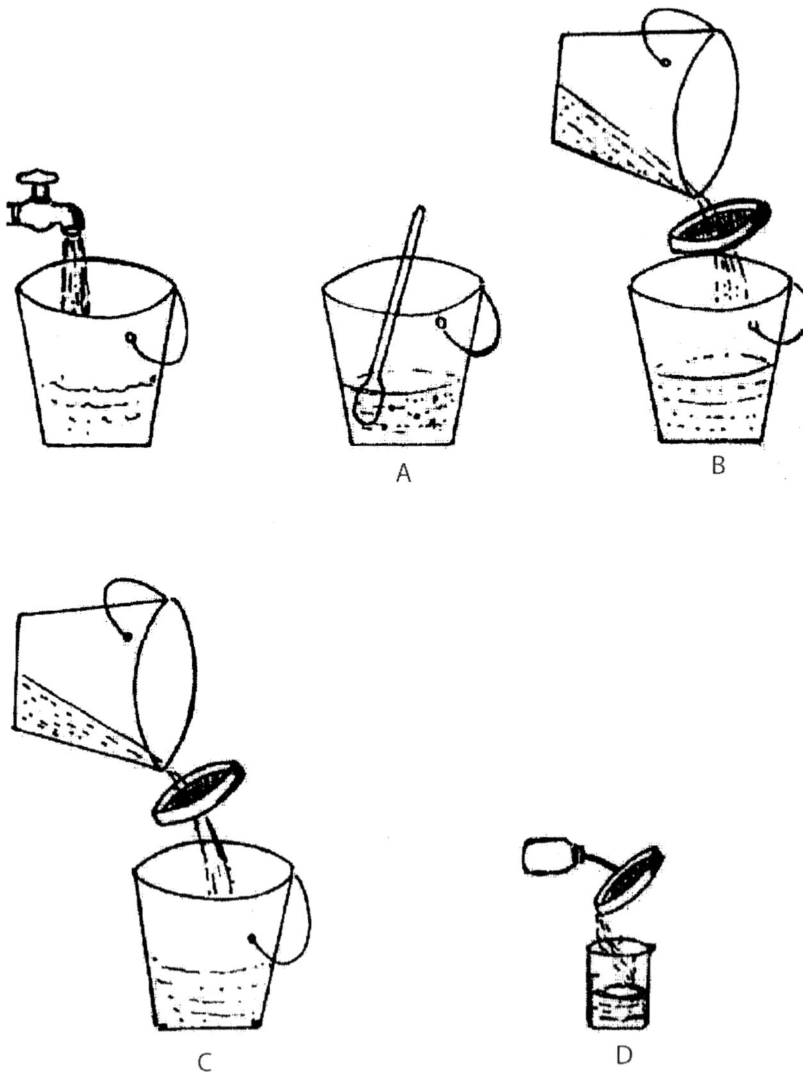

A. Soil in water is stirred thoroughly; **B.** Suspension passed through 20 mesh sieve; **C.** Nematodes are caught in 350 mesh sieve; **D.** Nematodes caught are transferred to a 250ml plastic beaker using a squeeze bottle

Fig. 13: Cobb's decanting and sieving method

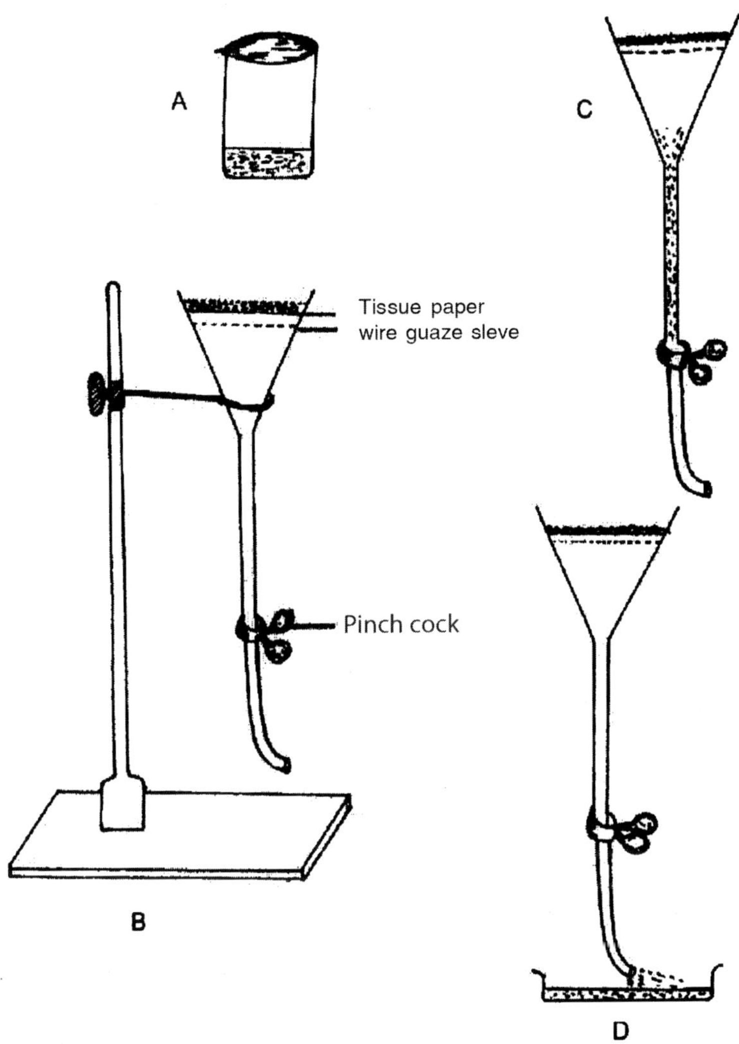

A. Beaker with soil and nematode in water suspension; **B.** Funnel assembly with nematode soil suspension poured over the tissue paper; **C.** Nematode sinking down the funnel tube; **D.** Nematode are collected in a Petri dish after 12 hours

Fig. 14: Baermann's funnel method

Precautions

Care should be taken to ensure that no nematode is lost by over flowing or spilling or splashing while transferring from one basin to another. In general, this method works better with sandy and sandy loam soils. The suspension can be poured efficiently if the sieves are agitated gently while pouring.

Advantages

1. Yields clean, healthy nematode specimens for inoculation purposes.
2. Some genera such as *Trichodorus* and *Helicotylenchus* are readily yielded in large numbers.

Disadvantages

1. Does not always yield sluggish forms such as *Criconemoides*, *Criconema* and *Hemicriconemoides* even when these are abundant in the soil sample.
2. The tissue paper acts as a barrier for swollen females.
3. If the residues are dense and abundant such as from clay and silt, then the nematode activity is inhibited due to oxygen suppression.
4. Very fine soil particles sometimes pass through the tissue papers and making the sample difficult to observe.
5. Length of time involved is considerably more.

Simple extraction method for larger nematodes like *Xiphinema* and *Longidorus*

1. Mix 100 ml of soil with water in basin I. After stirring thoroughly, the supernatant is decanted into basin II.
2. After stirring, the suspension in basin II is poured over 100 mesh sieve.
3. The catch on 100 mesh sieve is transferred into a beaker.
4. The nematode suspension in the beaker is poured on to a wire gauze containing two layers of tissue paper kept in a Petri dish holding sufficient water to remain in contact with the bottom of the wire gauze.
5. The next day the nematodes can be collected in clear water in the Petri dish.

Two - flask Technique

This method is based on the principle of counter flow (Fig. 15). Place 500 ml of the soil sample in a basin with 700 ml of water. The resultant suspension is passed through a coarse sieve (to remove pieces of roots and stones) and poured into a 2 litres Erlenmeyer flask (A), which is filled with water and capped. After vigorous shaking, flask (A) is overturned and placed on a second Erlenmeyer flask (B) which has already been filled with water. The heavy particles of soil will settle in the lower flask (B) and displaced water pass into the upper flask (A). The counter flow in the first few minutes prevents the lighter soil particles and nematodes from settling. After approximately 10 minutes, flask (A) is removed from flask (B), agitated and placed for another 10 minutes in a Becher glass (C) filled with water. Flask (B) is likewise capped, overturned and placed in another Becher glass (D). Within 10 minutes (20 minutes from the commencement of the procedure) flask (a) is removed from the Becher glass (C) and flask (B) placed in it (C) for another 10 minutes. Both the flasks now contain small nematodes and soil particles less than 50 m in size, while the Becher glass (C) contains larger nematodes and soil particles less than 100 m in size. The sediment from both sieves is put aside while the contents of the Becher glass (D) are agitated, left to rest for a minute or two, then poured through a sieve with a 250 m aperture. This sediment is then combined with that from Becher glass (C) and both flasks are placed on a sieve with a cotton wool filter. The nematodes pass through the cotton wool filter and collect in the clear water.

Elutriation Techniques

Two elutriation systems are in use based on the principle that a measure flow of water in an upward direction will support nematodes in a given range of specific gravity but with a low heavier solid debris to pass downward so that the nematodes can be collected in a relatively clean state. Both the elutriation systems are similar in principle but differ markedly in that each requires specialized apparatus and processing methods peculiar to the system.

The use of the elutriation system at present is to secure nematodes for inoculation purposes and those nematode genera which are not readily yielded by sieving and decantation technique, such as *Criconemoides*, *Criconema* and *Hemicriconemoides*.

The Oostenbrink Elutriation System

The step-by-step procedure of this system is as follows:

1. Before starting, fill the apparatus with clean water until the outlet of the funnel (up to level 1) passes a constant water stream of 1000 ml/min. through a perforated pipe from the bottom of the can (Fig. 16).
2. Mix the soil thoroughly. A sample of 500 ml moist soil is placed in the 1 mm pore size top sieve.
3. Wash the sample into the can via the funnel by means of a nozzle delivering about 700 ml/min until two-thirds of the column is filled up to level 2.

4. Turn off the top nozzle, reduce the constant water stream from the bottom to 600 ml/min until the water reaches level 3.
5. The suspension is poured into 4 sieves of 350 mesh placed on top of one another.
6. The catch is immediately washed into a 250 ml beaker.
7. Transfer the nematode suspension on to a wire gauge containing two layers of tissue paper. Place the wire gauge with tissue paper in a Petri dish holding sufficient water to remain in contact with the bottom of the wire gauge.
8. Leave the Petri dish setup overnight (12 h). The final suspension containing the nematodes in the Petri dish will be ready for observation.

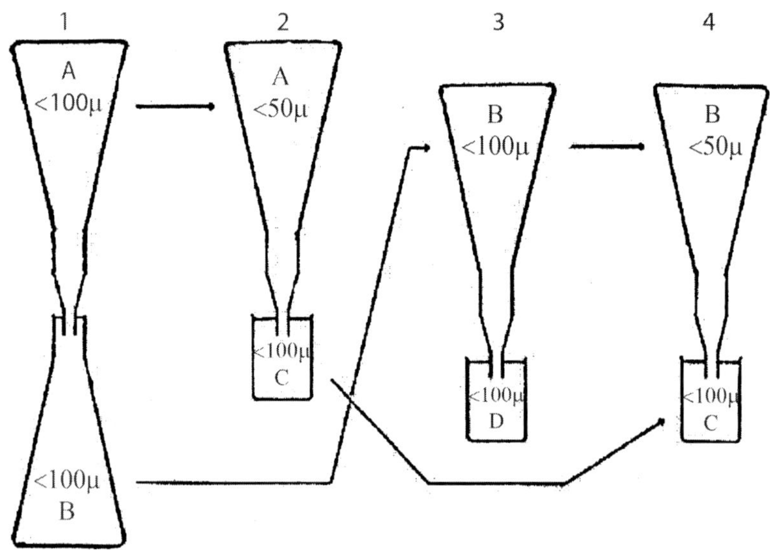

Fig. 15: Seinhorst's two-flask extraction technique

Centrifugal floatation technique

Nematodes can be extracted from soil and organic debris by floating them out in a solution with specific gravity greater than their own. As the method does not rely on the natural mobility of nematodes, it is extremely good for extracting even sluggish forms such as Criconematids, dead or fixed nematodes and nematode eggs. Centrifugal floatation is a generally more efficient nematode extraction method than modified Baermann's or elutriation techniques. This method is also often used to clean up the extracts obtained by sieving or elutriation. Solutions of sucrose, $MgSO_4$ or $ZnSO_4$ are usually used but nematodes may be distorted or even killed by osmotic stress and they should be rinsed with excess water after recovery in the sieve. Sugar solutions are extensively used since they are cheap and readily available.

In this method the floatation of nematodes was made possible with use of sugar solution of greater specific gravity (1.18) than that of the nematode (1.05).

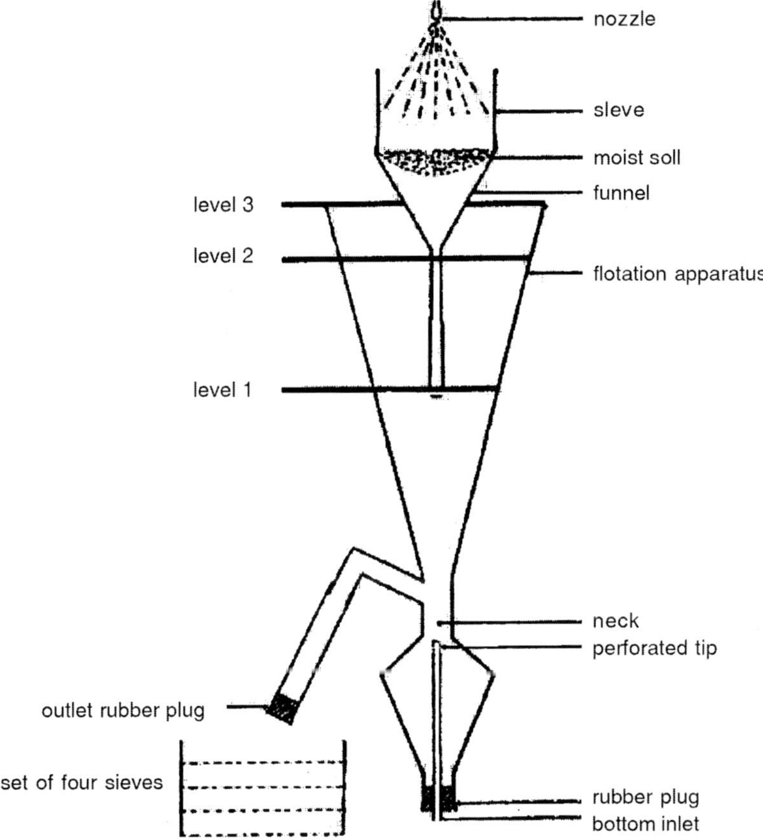

Fig. 16: Oostenbrink elutriation system for extraction of nematodes from soil

Materials required

1. Centrifuge
2. 350 mesh sieve
3. Sugar solution (1.18 Specific gravity)

The step-by-step procedure of this technique is as follows.

1. Transfer the suspension (obtained by decantation technique) to the centrifuge tubes distributing the contents equally between the tubes to maintain the balance and smooth running. Add water if needed to maintain uniform level in each tube and run the centrifuge at 3000 rpm for 4 minutes.
2. The nematodes and debris of nearly equal or greater specific gravity than that of the nematodes will be compacted at the bottom of the centrifuge tube. Discard the supernatant solution by slowly pouring off with a rotation motion of the hand so as to pour off most of the debris around the brim of the tube.
3. Refill the centrifuge tube with sugar solution (dissolve 484 g of sugar in water, add 10 ml of 10 per cent acetic acid to inhibit mould and bacterial growth and make up the volume to one litre) and run the centrifuge at 3000 rpm for two minutes.
4. Nematodes and debris of nearly equal specific gravity will be in the supernatant sugar solution. The soil and other debris will be compacted at the bottom of the tube.
5. Transfer the supernatant to a basin containing more quantity of water.
6. Pass the water in the basin through 350 mesh sieve by adding copious water to wash sugar solution from the nematode.
7. Gently flush the residues through the 350 mesh sieve into a 250 ml beaker using a squeeze bottle.

Precaution

Sugar solution causes damage to the nematodes. After the addition of sugar solution, further procedure needs to be done as quick as possible. After catching in 350 mesh sieve the nematodes must be exposed to sufficient amount of water to wash the sugar solution adhering to the cuticle.

Advantages

1. Quick method for extracting nematodes.
2. All types of soil are processed easily.
3. Nematode recovery is high.
4. Almost all genera can be obtained.

5. Swollen, sessile and sluggish nematodes can also be recovered.
6. Time schedule is relatively short.

Disadvantages

1. Sugar solution has got detrimental effect on the nematodes and hence the nematodes cannot be used for inoculation purpose.
2. Genera like *Trichodorus* and *Helicotylenchus* are obtained in lesser numbers.

Extraction of cysts from soil sample

1. Conical flask method

Principle

- Dry cysts lighter in weight, float in water and adhere to the sides of the container due to surface tension.

Procedure

- Collect the soil sample and shade dry.
- Transfer a known quantity of soil into a conical flask, add water and shake well.
- Add water up to the rim of the conical flask and leave it for 10 minutes.
- Cysts will float and get collected in the rim.
- Place a filter paper over a beaker and pour the suspension.
- Cysts will be retained in the filter paper.

Allow the filter paper to dry and examine under microscope.

Modified Fenwick Can Method

This Fenwick can apparatus is widely used for extraction of cysts from soil. This apparatus was developed by Fenwick in the year 1940. The can is usually made of brass of 30 cm height, tapering towards the top and have a sloping base. There is a drain hole of 2.5 cm diameter in the side of the can at the lowest point of the slope. Just below the rim of the can is a sloping collar with an upright rim of 6 cm height. The collar taper towards the outlet which is 4 cm wide. A large brass funnel 20.5 cm in diameter, with a stem 20.5 cm long, is supported above it and a 1mm aperture sieve fits into the funnel. The collecting sieves are placed below the outlet from the collar (Fig.17).

First fill the can with water and wet the collecting sieves. Place 100 ml of the prepared dry soil in the top sieve of 1 mm aperture. Wash the sample into the apparatus through the funnel. The coarse material is retained on top sieve. Heavy soil particles sink to the bottom of the can. The floating cysts are carried off over the overflow collar. The cysts along with minute dirts and root debris collected on 60 mesh sieve placed just below the overflow collar.

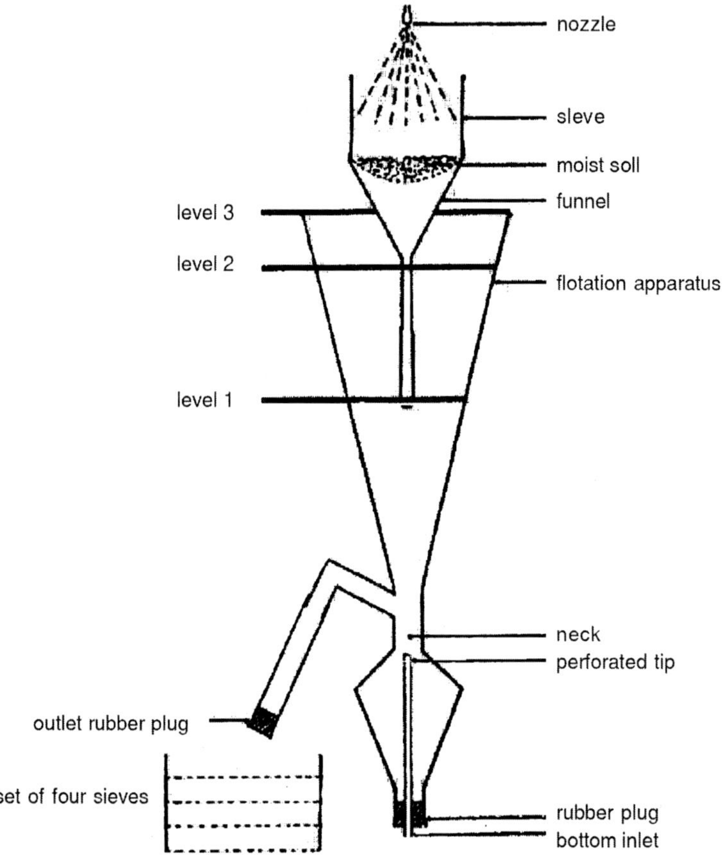

Fig. 17: Modified Fenwick can

The catch of the 60 mesh sieve is poured into a white bowl or basin. The cysts normally float along the edge of the bowl can be collected with a camel hair brush and counted. The cysts can be observed under the stereoscopic microscope using additional top focusing light.

Extraction of nematodes from roots and other plant materials

Extraction of nematodes from plant parts

Objective : To extract nematodes from plant parts for identification and estimation of population.

Methods

1. Direct examination

Procedure

1. Wash the infested plant material thoroughly and chop into small pieces
2. Put this material in a Petri dish containing water
3. Migratory and endo/semi endoparasitic nematodes that come out of the chopped material and move into water can be seen directly under microscope
4. Alternatively the chopped material can be processed by modified Baermann's funnel technique

2. Root incubation method

Principle

The nematodes migrate out of the roots due to suffocation

Procedure

1. Wash the roots to remove the adhering soil particles
2. Place the longitudinally cut wet roots in half of the polythene bag/glass jar
3. Seal the jar by screwing the lid with a few loose turns (do not tighten) or secure the polythene bag with rubber band
4. Incubate at 15°C for 72 h
5. Remove the nematodes, which have migrated out of the roots by flushing the roots with water for three times
6. Pass the washed water through 350-mesh sieve and collect the residue into a beaker with little water

3. Mechanical maceration or Waring blender or Homogenizer or Disintegrator technique

Principle

On maceration of the infested roots, the nematodes get separated from the root tissues because of mechanical force.

Procedure

1. Wash the roots with water to remove adhering soil particles
2. Chop the roots to 0.5-1.0 cm pieces and transfer them to a blender containing about 100 ml water (up to blade level)
3. Run the blender for 15 sec (30-60 sec for aged/hard roots)
4. Pour the resultant mixture into 60-mesh sieve followed by 350-mesh sieve and wash gently with a stream of water
5. Discard root residues in 60-mesh sieve and collect the nematode suspension on 350-mesh sieve in a beaker
6. Transfer the nematode suspension into modified Baermann's funnel.

Counting and picking of nematodes

Objective : To estimate the nematode population in a given suspension and to transfer nematodes from one solution to another while processing.

Nematode counting

Direct counting method

This method is used when the nematode population in the suspension is very low.

Procedure

1. Transfer the nematode suspension to a counting dish
2. Keep the counting dish under stereomicroscope
3. Adjust one small square of the counting dish from one side under microscope and record the number of nematodes using tally counter
4. Proceed to the next square and so on to count from all the squares.

Dilution method

This method is used when the nematode population in the suspension is very high.

Procedure

1. Take the nematode suspension in a beaker and make a volume of 100 ml by adding water and mix the suspension thoroughly
2. Transfer 5 ml of nematode suspension to a counting dish and count the nematodes as described above
3. Repeat this procedure 3 times
4. Calculate the average number of nematodes per 5 ml
5. Multiply with 20 (5ml x 20 = 100ml) to calculate the total number of nematodes present in the sample.

Picking of nematodes

1. Take the nematode suspension in a cavity block or Petri dish and focus the nematode under a low magnification of stereomicroscope
2. Lift the nematode to the surface of the water while focusing along the floating nematode
3. Flick the nematode quickly up so that the nematode is pulled out through the meniscus

Staining and Histopathological Techniques

Investigation of host-parasite relationship involving endoparasitic nematodes requires use of methods that faciliate observation of nematodes inside roots. Limited information may be obtained simply by the staining of nematodes. They need to be observed in the interior tissues of roots. For more detailed studies of host-parasite relationship, infected roots may be prepared by histological methods and sectioned before examination.

Staining nematodes in plant tissue

Study on endoparasitic species often involves study of the penetration and development of specimens within intact roots. Many procedures for staining and clearing nematode-infected plant tissues have been developed and most of these are satisfactory for various kinds of tissues. The acidfuchsin-lactophenol method, developed in 1941, has been the most widely used procedure.

However, two other procedures which are noteworthy as being very reliable, relatively simple to use and superior to the acidfuchsin-lactophenol method are as follows.

Sodium hypochlorite-acid fuchsin method

This new method for clearing and staining nematode infected root tissues has several advantages over other procedures. First, it eliminates exposure of personnel to toxic substances like phenol which are utilized in other methods. The root tissue is cleared with sodium hypochlorite (NaOCl) prior to staining with acid fuchsin, it will not become heavily stained. As a result, the time required for destaining is shortened and frequent destaining is unnecessary. This method is excellent for staining endoparasitic nematodes in soybean and cotton roots. The tissue-clearing step (treatment with NaOCl) may need to be modified slightly for roots of other plant species.

The step-by-step procedure is as follows.

1. Wash infected roots and place them in a 150 ml beaker. The roots are cut into segments or stained intact; however, large root systems could be cut into sections for staining.
2. Clear the roots by adding 50 ml of tap water plus an appropriate amount of chlorine bleach (5.25% NaOCl). The amount of bleach needed depends on the age of the root tissue. The following suggestions are guidelines for the quantity of bleach to be added.

   Young roots - add 10 ml 5.25% NaOCl

   Moderate-age roots - add 20 ml 5.25% NaOCl

   Older or more ligneous roots- add 20 ml 5.25% NaOCl
3. Soak roots for 4 minutes in the NaOCl solution and agitate occasionally.
4. Rinse roots for approximately 45 seconds in running tap water then soak them in tap water for 15 minutes to remove any residual NaOCl which may affect staining with acid fuchsin.
5. Drain the water and transfer roots to a beaker with 30-50 ml of tap water.
6. Add one ml of stock acid-fuchsin-stain solution to the water. (Stock solution is prepared by dissolving 3.5 g acid fuchsin in 250 ml acetic acid and 750 ml distilled water).
7. Boil the solution for about 30 seconds on a hot plate or in a microwave oven.

8. Cool the solution to room temperature, drain it from the roots and rinse the roots in running tap water.
9. Place roots in 20-30 ml of glycerin acidified with a few drops of HCl and heat to boiling for destaining.
10. Following the destaining process, roots may be either stored in acidified glycerin with little change in contrast between nematodes and root tissue.

Lactophenol method

This method has been the most widely used method in the staining of nematodes in plant tissue. Infected roots of young plants or small roots of older plants, respond best to this technique. This staining technique is apparently not suitable for roots with a high fat content such as most perennials, since their roots will retain too much of the stain. The disadvantage of this procedure is that the destaining processes not easily regulated and often takes several days. The process is accelerated when stained roots are placed in clear lactophenol and autoclaved for 10 minutes at 15 lb pressure.

Procedure

1. Prepare lactophenol by mixing liquid phenol, lactic acid, glycerin and distilled water in the ratio of 1:1:2:1.
2. Prepare stain solution by adding 5 ml of 1% stock solution of acid fuchsin or cotton blue per 100 ml of lactophenol. The concetration of stain may need to be varied depending on the age of tissue used for the study.
3. Add stain to a beaker and boil on a hot plate. Immerse infected roots in boiling stain for about 1 minute, rinse them in tap water and destain in clear lactophenol solution until maximum contrast between the nematodes and root tissue is obtained. The solution may be heated in a water bath (100°C) or an oven (70°C) for about 90 to 120 minutes to avoid direct boiling. Destaining usually requires from a few hours upto several days.

Counting nematodes in root tissue

Stained endoparasitic nematodes may be counted directly in intact root tissue or following root maceration technique.

Direct counting

Roots are easily examined when distributed in a small amount of glycerin on a Petri dish cover or a transparent plastic counting dish and pressed against the cover with the Petri dish bottom. Marking a grid on the Petri dish aids in counting the nematodes under a stereoscopic microscope

Extracting nematodes

Considerable time is required for direct counting of nematodes inside large root systems. Nematodes, however, can be freed from the roots by maceration and a sub sample can be removed for counting. Roots may be macerated in a warring blender. Nematodes can be separated from the root tissue by sieving. However, care must be taken to ensure that nematodes are not ruptured or destained during maceration.

Methods of microtechnique in nematology

Histological studies involving endoparasitic nematodes required to prepare thin sections of infected root tissues with a minimum distortion. The examination of such sections with the microscope can be used to study and compare the reactions of various tissues to nematodes. Tissues embedded in a matrix of either paraffin wax or plastic blocks will be easily sectioned and handled. The sectioning of paraffin-embedded tissue requires less sophisticated equipment and a greater quantity of tissue may be more rapidly examined. However, thinner sections can be cut from plastic-embedded tissue and greater cytologic details may be observed. The following steps are required in the preparation of materials for histopathological study with the paraffin wax method.

Tissue selection and preparation

Samples of healthy and infected root tissues should be included in all histopathological studies. It is also often advisable to collect infected tissues at different stages of nematode development. Roots must be dug, not pulled out from the plant. Wash the roots gently and thoroughly under running tap water to remove soil particles. Even a small particle of soil adhering to the tissues will damage the microtome knife during sectioning. Tissues should be cut into smaller pieces and placed into a container of fixative as soon as possible. Small roots should be cut with a sharp razor blade into lengths of about 1 cm while immersed in a drop of water. Large roots and stems (greater than 1 cm diameter) should also be cut longitudinally for a better exchange of chemicals during processing. When tissues are prepared for fixation, care must always be taken that the tissue is not crushed or allowed to desiccate during handling.

Fixation

Fixation kills the nematode and also preserves the cellular structures. One of the best and most common fixatives is formalin-acetoalcohol (FAA) which is a mixture of 90 ml of 50% ethanol, 5 ml of glacial acetic acid and 5 ml of 37% formaldehyde. Another fixative that works well in formalin propiono-propanol (FPP) which is a mixture of 90 ml of 50% isopropyl alcohol, 5 ml of propionic acid and 5 ml of 37% formaldehyde. The proportions of reagents given for FAA and FPP are satisfactory and may be varied for certain types of materials, if poor results are obtained with the standard concentrations.

In fixation, the tissue should be submerged in a volume of fixative at least 10 times greater than that of the volume of the tissue to ensure that the fixative does not become over diluted by water from the tissue. If pieces do not sink rapidly into the fixative, the container of fixative may be placed under a mild vacuum to draw air out of the tissue more quickly. Tissue must remain in the fixative for a minimum of 24 hr to several days, depending on its thickness. Materials can also be stored indefinitely in the fixative.

Dehydration

Dehydration removes water from the tissue. Water must be removed gradually to avoid plasmolysis. Therefore, dehydration is accomplished by moving the tissue stepwise through increasing higher concentrations of alcohol. When FAA is used as the fixative, the tertiary-butyl-alcohol (TBA) dehydration schedule should be followed (Table.1). If the material has been fixed in FPP, the isopropyl-alcohol (IPA) dehydration schedule should be followed (Table 2).

When solutions in the dehydration schedule are changed, the liquid is drained from the container holding the tissue and then the tissue is covered immediatedly with the next solution. Care must be taken that the material is never allowed to desiccate. The time required for the material to remain in the various dehydrating solutions depends on its thickness. For example, fine roots may need minimum length of time, whereas thick woody material requires maximum length of time.

Infiltration

In this step, alcohol in the tissues are replaced by paraffin wax so that the tissue is saturated with a pure solution of paraffin. When the TBA dehydration schedule has been followed, the 100% TBA solution after step 8 is first replaced with 1:1 mixture of 100% TBA and paraffin oil. The tissue is allowed to remain in this solution for 1 hr or more, depending on its thickness. Shortly before the next step, another container is filled with melted paraffin upto 3/4 of its volume and the paraffin is allowed to solidify slightly. The tissue in the TBA paraffin oil mixture is then placed on top of the solidified paraffin and is covered with a layer of TBA paraffin oil solution.

Table.1: Tertiary butyl alcohol dehydration schedule.

Quantity (ml) needed for solution						
Step	% Alcohol	Time	Distilled Water	95% ethanol	100% ethanol	100% TBA
1	50	2 hr or more	50	40	0	10
2	70	Overnight	30	50	0	20
3	85	1-2 hr	15	50	0	35
4	95	1-2 hr	0	45	0	55
5	100	1-3 hr	0	0	25	75
6	100	1-3 hr	0	0	0	100
7	100	1-3 hr	0	0	0	100
8	100	Overnight	0	0	0	100

Table 2: Isopropyl alcohol dehydration schedule.

Quantity (ml) needed for solution				
Step	%Alcohol	Time	Distilled Water	100% IBA
1	70	1 day - 1 wk	30	70
2	90	1 day - 1 wk	10	90
3	100	1 day - 1 wk	0	100
4	100	1 day - 1 wk	0	100

This container is placed uncovered in an oven that is set slightly above the melting point of the paraffin. The tissue sinks to the bottom of the container as the paraffin melts. After 1 to 3 hr the TBA paraffin oil-paraffin mixture is poured off and replaced with pure melted paraffin.

The uncovered container is then placed back in the oven for about 3 hr. This step should be repeated at least once. Next, the melted paraffin is replaced by a specialized type of paraffin, specially made for histological use. Tissue should remain in the paraffin for 12 hr or overnight in an oven.

The infiltration procedure to be followed when the IPA dehydration schedule has been used is much simpler but requires a greater length of time. First, part of the 100% IPA in the last dehydration step is poured off so that the tissue in the bottom of the container remains covered. The container is then filled with chips of wax and is placed uncovered in an oven set at 59-60°C. Once the chips have melted, the paraffin-IPA mixture is poured off and replaced with pure melted wax. This paraffin should be exchanged for freshly melted wax twice at 3 to 4 day interval. Small, fine roots should be ready to embed 1 week after beginning of the infiltration procedure while thicker tissue may take 1 to 2 weeks to embed in the wax.

Embedding

In embedding, the tissue is positioned in cooling paraffin so that it can be sectioned after hardening. Moulds for embedding may either be constructed in the lab out of folded paper or metal base moulds and embedding rings designed especially for histology may be purchased. Moulds should first be coated with a thin layer of glycerine. The sample is then poured or carefully lifted into the mould with heated forceps and additional melted paraffin is added to fill the mould. This step may be done on a hot plate set at 60°C. However, an embedding table, consisting of a rectangular metal plate which has a heat source at one end and which becomes progressively cooler toward the other end, gives increased control of the embedding procedure. The filled mould is next moved to a cooler surface either on the laboratory bench or on the embedding table. As soon as the paraffin begins to solidify on the bottom of the mould, the tissue is rapidly oriented in the desired fashion with a heated dissecting needle. Once the paraffin begins to solidify over the top of the mould, the mould is plunged into ice water and left there until the paraffin is completely solidified. After hardening, the paraffin is removed from the mould and may be cut into smaller blocks which can either be mounted on wooden blocks with melted paraffin or inserted directly into the microtome. Sample of tissue may be stored in these blocks indefinitely in a cool place.

Sectioning

Sectioning of paraffin blocks is done on a rotary microtome equipped with a knife or disposable razor blade. A knife must be used when the tissue is tough or woody. However, for other types of tissues, razor blades will cut sections equal in quality to the knife-cut sections. Because razor blades can be frequently replaced with fresh blades, they have the advantage of not requiring sharpening and therefore are useful when working with root tissue, which often carries solid particles that can rapidly dull a cutting edge.

Excess paraffin surrounding the tissue should be trimmed away before sectioning, leaving at least 1 mm around the tissue. Care should be taken so that the opposite edges of the trimmed block face are parallel. The block is then cooled in ice water for at least 5 minutes, inserted into the microtome clamp and one edge of its face aligned parallel to the knife edge. Sections of 8-12 m in thickness are usually taken for histological studies. Tissue that is especially tough or woody will section more easily if the trimmed block is first soaked overnight in the refrigerator in a softening solution consisting of 90 ml of 1% sodium lauryl sulphate and 10 ml of glycerine. The excess paraffin on the face of the block must first be trimmed away, exposing the tissue so that the softening solution can penetrate.

As the sections are cut, the edge of each section should adhere to the previous section to form a ribbon. A sharp knife edge and proper knife angle are most important in obtaining a ribbon. The back of the knife edge should also be checked frequently and cleaned if necessary as paraffin buildup will adversely affect ribbon formation. As the ribbon increases in length, it should be held away from the microtome with a dissecting needle or brush. It is then removed from the knife edge with a second needle and transferred to a clean, flat surface. The ribbon should never be touched with hands. The ribbons can either be mounted immediately or stored in a cool, dust-free place for several weeks if necessary.

Ribbon Mounting

Ribbon mounting adheres sections to glass microscope slides so that they can be stained. Ribbons must first be cut into shorter lengths so that they can be fit on to the slides. Slides may be labelled with a diamond pencil or if the glass on one end is frosted, with a lead pencil. The surface of the slides is then coated with a small amount of Haupt's adhesive which consists of 1g powdered high-grade gelatin, 100 ml distilled water, 2 g phenol crystals, and 15 ml glycerine. For preparation of the adhesive, the gelatin is dissolved in the water at 30°C, the phenol and glycerin are added and the solution is filtered. Before the adhesive dries on the slides, the slides are flooded with a 2-3% formalin solution, which should be made fresh each day. The flooded slides are then placed on a warming tray held at 25 to 30°C and segments of the ribbon are floated on the slides. As the slides warm up, the ribbon will flatten out and the liquid will evaporate. After several hours, when the slides are completely dry, they can be removed and stored indefinitely.

Staining

The process of staining removes the paraffin from the sections and increases the contrast in the tissue. Three staining procedures that have been used for nematode infected root materials are Johansen's Quadruple Stain (Table.3). Sass Safranin and Fast Green Stain (Table.4), and Triarch Quadruple Stain (Table.5).

Solutions made from dry, powdered stains should always be filtered before they are first used. If only a few slides are being stained, the alcohol and staining solutions may be kept in Couplin jars and the slides moved individually after each time period. However, larger containers and racks that hold 25 or 50 slides are more convenient when staining larger quantities. Stains and alcohol that are not being used over long periods should be stored in tightly capped bottles.

In these three staining schedules (Tables 3, 4 & 5), containers holding water rinses should be emptied and refilled with fresh water after each group of slides. Rinses containing alcohol should be changed when the liquid becomes heavily stained. Staining solutions and xylene often require replacement.

Table 3: Johansen's quadruple stain.

Step	Solution	Time
1	Xylene	5 min
2	Xylene-absolute ethanol (1:1)	5 min
3	95% ethanol	5 min
4	70% ethanol	5 min
5	Safranin O solution*	6-24hr
6	Rinse in tap water	
7	1% aqueous methyl violet 2B	10-15min
8	Rinse in tap water	
9	95% ethanol-methyl cellosolve-tertiary butyl alcohol (1:1:1)	15 sec
10	Fast green FCF solution**	10-15 min
11	95% ethanol-tertiary butyl alcohol (1:1)	
	plus 0.5% glacial acetic acid	15 sec
12	Orange G solution ***	3 min
13	Clove oil-methyl cellosolve 95%ethanol (1:1:1)	16 sec
14	Clove oil-absolute ethanol-xylene(1:1:1)	15 sec
15	Xylene	5 min
16	Xylene	5 min or longer

*The safranin O solution is prepared by dissolving 4g safranin O in 200 ml methyl cellosolve. When the safranin is dissolved, add 100 ml 95% ethanol and 100 ml distilled water. Finally, add 4g sodium acetate and 8 ml formalin.

Table 4: Sass safranin and fast green stain.

Step	Solution	Time
1	Xylene	5 min
2	Absolute ethanol	5 min
3	95% ethanol	5 min
4	70% ethanol	5 min
5	50% ethanol	5 min
6	30% ethanol	5 min
7	1% aqueous safranin O	1-12 hr
8	Rinse in tap water	
9	30% ethanol	3 min
10	50% ethanol	3 min
11	70% ethanol	3 min
12	95% ethanol	3 min
13	0.1% fast green FCG in 95% ethanol	5-30 sec

Step	Solution	Time
14	Absolute ehanol	15 sec
15	Absolute ehanol	3 min
16	Xylene-absolute ethanol	5 min
17	Xylene	5 min
18	Xylene	5 min or longer

Table 5: Johansen's quadruple stain.

Step	Solution	Time
1	Xylene	5 min
2	Xylene	5 min
3	Xylene-absolute ethanol (1:1)	5 min
4	95% ethanol	5 min
5	70% ethanol	5 min
6	1% safranin O in 50% ethanol	5-15 min
7	Rinse in distilled water	
8	1% aqueous crystal violet	1-2 min
9	Rinse in distilled water	
10	Absolute ehanol	30 sec
11	Absolute ehanol	30 sec
12	* Orange G-fast green ** (135 ml - 15 ml)	3 min
13	Orange G-fast green (145 ml - 5 ml)	2 min
14	Orange G-fast green (148 ml - 2 ml)	2 min
15	Orange G	2 min
16	Absolute ethanol	1 min
17	Xylene	5 min
18	Xylene	5 min or longer

**The fast green FCF solution is prepared by adding 0.25 g fast green FCG to 50 ml of a solution composed of methyl cellosolve and clove oil (1:1). After the fast green has dissolved, 150 ml 95% ethanol, 150 ml tertiary butyl alcohol and 3.5 ml glacial acetic acid are added.

***The orange G solution is prepared by dissolving 1g orange G in 200 ml methyl cellosolve and then adding 100 ml 95% ethanol.

*Orange G is prepared dissolving 0.4 g orange G in 100 ml clove oil.

**Fast green is prepared by dissolving 1g fast green FCF in 100 ml absolute ethanol.

After completion of staining procedure, coverslip are mounted with a few drops of either Canada balsum or DPX mountant. Slides are first removed from the xylene, which is always the final step in the staining procedure and laid on a flat absorbent surface. The mounting medium is then applied to the surface of the slide. A minimum of mounting medium should be used, as any excess will run out over the surface of the coverslip. Finished slides should be left flat to dry for at least 24 hr at room temperature. However, the medium will harden better if the slides are held on a 60°C warming tray overnight.

Stains turn lignified or cutinized cell walls as red whereas the fast green generally turns cellulose walls as greenish. Starch grains stain purple by methyl violet and crystal violet. Nemotodes in tissue vary from brownish to red. Triarch Quadruple Stain gives the best contrast consistently and takes the least amount of time. Also, a wide variety of tissue types may be stained without altering the staining time. However, since it requires a large amount of clove oil, it is the most expensive stain to prepare. Staining times in the Johansen's Quadruple Stain and Sass Safranin and Fast Green Stain may need to be adjusted for the best contrast between cell types.

Preparation of perineal patterns of *Meloidogyne* spp. for observation

Several methods have been described for preparation of perineal patterns. Some techniques involve fixation and staining of root material prior to removal of females, but Taylor & Netscher's procedure utilizes fresh root material, thereby eliminating exposure of eggs to toxic fixatives. Staining is necessary since it does not enhance the clarity of the diagnostic details of perineal patterns. Perineal patterns can be prepared from fresh root material that has been stored upto several weeks in a refrigerator.

The following materials are useful in the preparation of perineal patterns: a small surgical eye knife or single edged razor blade, forceps, half spear or teasing needle, pulp canal file, 45% lactic acid, glycerine, plastic Petri dish, syracuse dish, clean microscope slides, cover slip and sealing compound.

1. Select galls with mature females. Place in syracuse dish with tap water. Single galls are preferable than that of compound galls.
2. Tease the root tissue apart with forceps and half spear to remove adult females.
3. Rupture the cuticle of the female near the neck and gently push the body tissues out.
4. Place the cuticle in a drop of 45% lactic acid on a plastic Petri dish. The lactic acid facilitates the removal of body tissues that adhere to the cuticle after trimming. Collect 10 to 20 cuticles in a drop of lactic acid and let them stand for 30 minutes to several hours. All cuts with the eye knife are done on the surface of a plastic petri dish to minimize the damage to the knife. The knife can be re-sharpened with a fine-grit sharpening stone.
5. Cut the cuticle in half (equatorially) with cataract knife. Remove the cuticle with the perineal pattern from the drop of 45% lactic acid. Place

it next to the drop and trim the perineal pattern to a square. Place the trimmed perineal pattern back in the 45% lactic acid. Cut 5 to 10 perineal patterns per sample.

6. Thoroughly clean debris from the perineal pattern.
7. Transfer the perineal patterns to a drop of glycerine on a clean glass microscope slide. Align the perineal patterns so that they are in a straight line and the anus is oriented down. The interior surface of the cuticle must be placed against the glass. Press the perineal pattern gently against the glass with the pulp canal file.
8. Gently place the coverslip on the glycerine drop. Excess glycerine can be absorbed by a piece of filter paper. If there is insufficient glycerine under the coverslip, a small drop can be placed on the edge of the coverslip.
9. Seal the coverslip and label the slide. (Fig. 18).

Use of Microscopes in Nematology

Two types of microscopes are commonly used in the Nematological laboratory. They are the compound microscope and the stereoscopic microscope.

The best performance can be obtained only when the eyepieces, objectives, condenser and light source are accurately aligned with the axis of the body tube and the focusing racks of the condenser and body tube or stage are parallel with one another and with the tube axis. The bulb, collecting lens and the diaphragm of the lamp must be aligned with the optical axis.

Factors affecting the performance of the microscope alignment

Alignment of the objective with the eyepiece can be checked quickly after centering and checking alignment of the condenser, lamp and mirror. With proper alignment, the image of the lamp iris viewed through microscope fitted with high power objective should have a uniform colour fringe. Diversity of colour suggests misalignment which may be due to an inaccurate fit to a poor objective.

Objectives

Of the objectives for normal microscopic, photomicrography and apochromates of largest numerical aperture give best central resolution and contrast. They are generally the best objectives for critical visual examination of fine detail.

Numerical aperture

Objectives are rated not only by their power of magnification, but also by their numerical aperture. The numerical aperture of an objective is almost directly proportional to its resolving power and is defined by the following equation.

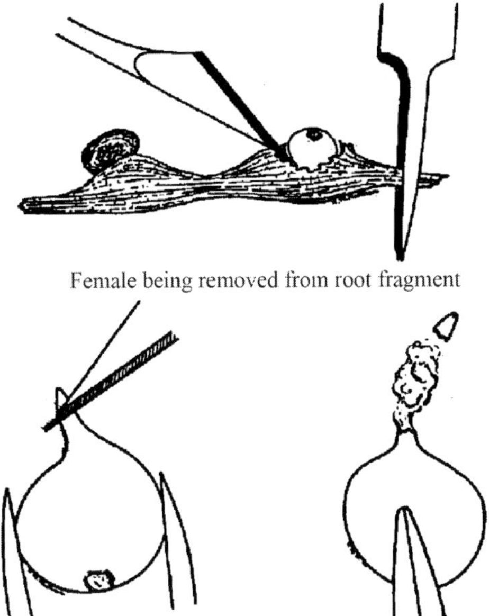

Female being removed from root fragment

Cuticle being trimmed around the perineal pattern

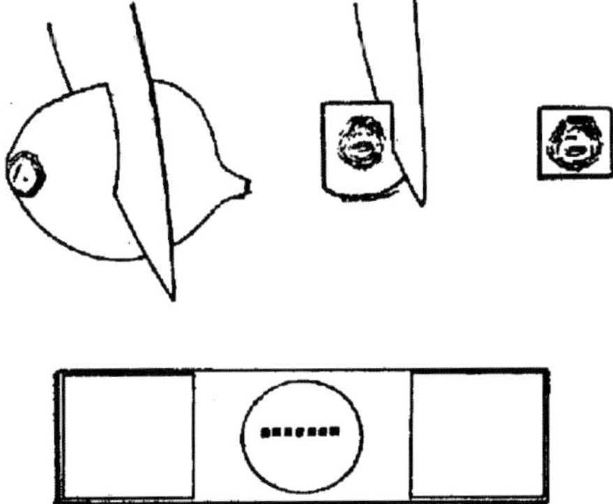

Exposed female being ruptured and body tissues gently removed

Fig. 18: Preparation of perineal pattern of *Meloidogyne* spp.

Where n is the refractive index of the medium between object and objective and U is the angle of aperture. U is thoretically 90° when the objective is touching the object. Therefore the numerical aperture of a dry lens cannot exceed 1.0 (n=1; sin 90° = 1); in practice 0.95 is about the greatest that can be achieved.

Oil-immersion objectives

If immersion oil (n=1.5) is placed between object and objective the highest theoretical numerical aperture is 1.5 sin 90° = 1.5. In practice the maximum which can be achieved is about 1.45 and most oil immersion objectives have numerical aperture = 1.25-1.3. Mostly the oil immersion objectives are with the magnification of 100 x. Great care is needed while focusing, because of very small working distance which is usually less than 1 mm. It is therefore important to use correct cover-glass thickness.

Stereomicroscope

A wide range of excellent stereoscopic microscopes are available. The most important features are a wide flat field, good and even transmitted light source with excellent resolution.

General care to be taken while using the microscopes

Clean optical components are essential, but wrong cleaning methods damage them. Dirt should be prevented from reaching optical parts. Cleaning should be gentle and minimal. Locate dirt spots by rotating optical components in turn, while viewing an illuminated field with a small substage-iris aperture. When the spots move, remove and clean the component. Use only special lens tissues for wiping, after breathing on the glass and rigidly follow the rule, 'one tissue, one wipe'; remove dry dusts with a bulb-type blower or compressed air. Tenacious grease marks may be dissolved with a little ether preferably applied to all but the edge of the lens with a soft, clean brush. Before evaporation, remove the solvent by a single, light circular wipe with a lens tissue covering at any moment at least the full radius of the lens. Clean very small lenses in sunk mounts by first twirling a wisp of cotton wool round a sharpened matchstick to make a small 'bud', then wrapping the 'bud' in a lens tissue and using the same wiping action as before. Moistening the bud in solvent directly or using a tissue for more than one wipe only leaves worse smears.

Objectives of high power and high NA are especially susceptible to damage because of the thinness of metal required to support the front lens. Great care in focusing them is essential.

Do's and dont's while handling microscopes

- Untrained operators must not be allowed to use the microscopes and laboratory for work with nematodes.
- Ideally, the high-power microscopes should be permanently installed on a flat vibration-free bench away from corrosive chemicals and vapours.
- To minimise the risk of damage, move and carry microscopes as little as possible.
- When moving and carrying the instrument be sure that it is securely held and take care.
- Replace dust covers immediately after use and when appropriate return the instrument to its cabinet.
- Liquids split on the instrument should be removed with a soft cloth or lens tissue as soon as possible. Immersion oil should be removed from oil-immersion lenses, other lenses and microscope slides by means of lens tissue only.
- Never lubricate moving parts unless with a specified lubricant. If you are uncertain about a suitable lubricant, contact the manufacturer's representative or a reputable service engineer.
- Avoid touching lenses with fingers.
- Marks on lenses should be removed by wiping with a disposable lens tissue, if necessary moistened with a solvent approved by the manufacturer.
- Never dismantle objectives and condensers.
- Dust on the back of objectives and condensers and dismantles eyepieces only if the inside surface of lenses need cleaning.
- Remove dust from outer lens surface by blowing with a rubber bulb or compressed air or wiping with a lens tissue.
- Never touch the surface of internal prisms, if they are dusty blow them with a rubber bulb or compressed air.
- Keep additional and spare optical components in a robust container in a secure place.
- Focus by racking initially so that the objective and object move apart. It is useful to mark on the focusing drive which direction separates stages from objective.

- Indicate on the base of the microscope which objectives need immersion oil (60-65 x may be dry or oil). Do not go back to high-power dry objectives (40-65 x) when oil is on the slide.
- After the use, remove the specimen and place the lowest power objective in the optical axis.
- Do not keep the microscope lamp burning longer than necessary. Remember that, with a variable transformer, using the lamp beyond the normal intensity range for a prolonged period will severely reduce its life.
- Do not touch the glass of quartz-halogen bulbs.
- Have the instrument serviced annually either by the manufacture's representative or by reputable service engineer. If it is not functioning correctly contact the manufacturer's representative.

Observing Slide with the nematode specimen in the Microscope

- Place the object on stage.
- Adjust the reflector so that light beam is transmitted on to the object.
- Focus the object by moving focusing knob.
- For viewing under high magnification either move the objective or change the magnification changer.

2. Compound microscope

Purpose

- To study the morphological characters of nematodes at higher magnification (40X to 100X)

Parts

- Base: having empty space for the attachment of a lamp and / or a reflector mirror
- Condenser: with condenser lens, an aperture diaphragm, filter holder and a knob for its movement
- Rectangular object stage with clips for holding slide and coaxial knobs for the movement of the slide
- Knobs for coarse and fine focusing

- Revolving nose piece with objective of 4X, 10X, 40X and 100X; 100X objective lens is also known as oil immersion lens because when we use this lens, immersion oil ($\mu = 1.515$) is placed over the cover slip
- Neck of the microscope
- Binocular ocular tube with eye pieces of 10X or 15X and adjustment for inter-pupillary distance

Handling

- Place the slide on the stage and secure it with clips.
- Focus under 4X objective with a coarse focusing knob. Then use fine adjustment knobs for exact focusing.
- Move the condenser lens and adjust diaphragm to control contrast.
- For viewing under immersion oil lens first focus under 4X or 10X lens.
- Move the nose piece. Put a drop of immersion oil on the coverslip and then focus under 100X lens, using a fine focusing knob.

Differences between stereoscopic and compound microscopes

Sl.No	Stereoscopic microscope	Compound microscope
1.	Magnification is low (usually less than 70X)	Magnification is high (usually 40X – 100X)
2.	Working distance is high	Working distance is low
3.	Three dimensional image is formed	Three dimensional image is not formed
4.	Erect image is formed	Inverted image is formed

Preservation, processing and mounting of nematode specimens

a. Killing of nematodes

Small samples

- Place a drop of water on a glass slide and transfer few nematodes from the suspension using a pick.
- Show the slide over a flame for 5-6 seconds or add two drops of hot water to a drop of water containing the nematodes.

Large sample

- Concentrate the nematode suspension to a small quantity in a vial.
- Plunge the vial in hot water at 60°C in a beaker for 2 minutes.

b. Fixing of nematodes

- Take the concentrated nematode suspension in a screw cap vial and add equal quantity of hot fixative.
- Label the vials with the name of nematode, source of collection, fixative used, date of collection and date of fixation. Vial containing fixed specimen in fixative is called wet collection.

Fixatives

FA 4:1

Formalin (40% formaldehyde) – 10 ml

Glacial acetic acid – 1 ml

Distilled water – 89 ml

TAF

Formalin (40% formaldehyde) – 7 ml

Triethanolamine – 2ml

Distilled water – 91 ml

Formalin 4%

Formalin – 4 ml

Distilled water – 96 ml

FAA

Ethanol 95% – 20ml

Formalin – 6ml

Glacial acetic acid – 1ml

Distilled water – 40ml

c. Processing

Processing of nematode specimens clears the internal body contents of the fixed nematodes and makes clearly visible. Specimens can be processed with lactophenol, lactoglycerol or glycerol, which also serve as suitable mountant.

1. Lactophenol method

- Fill cavity slide with lactophenol (phenol liquid - 1 part, lactic acid - 1 part, glycerol - 2 parts, distilled water - 1 part) and heat on a hot plate at 65°C.
- Transfer the fixed nematode specimens to lactophenol when it is hot and allow for 2-3 minutes.

2. Slow method or Glycerol method

- Transfer the specimens from fixative to 2 ml of 1.5% glycerol in distilled water in a small watch glass or cavity block.
- Add a trace amount of picric acid or copper sulphate to prevent mould growth.
- Place the watch glass or cavity block in a desiccator for about 4 weeks.

3. Rapid method or Seinhorst's method

Seinhorst's solution I

96% ethanol – 20 ml

Glycerol – 1 ml

Distilled water – 79 ml

Seinhorst's solution II

Glycerol – 5 parts

96% ethanol – 95 parts

- Transfer the fixed specimens to a cavity block containing 1/3 volume with Seinhorst solution I.
- Place the cavity block on a platform support or grid in a dessicator filled 96% ethanol at the bottom and keep at room temperature.
- After 12 hours, carefully remove the excess ethonal using ink filler or hypodermic syringe. Specimens should not be disturbed while removing.

- Add few drops of Seinhorst solution II into cavity block and leave slight opening of lid.
- Place in a dessicator containing calcium chloride at the bottom and keep at room temperature
- Remove the specimens using pick and mount them after three days. Specimens will be in pure anhydrous glycerine after processing.

Note

Bigger specimens like *Hoplolaimus* and *XIphinema* will collapse if the cavity block lid is opened partially or more solution is added due to rapid loss of ethonal,

Baker's method

- Place a drop of Baker's solutions I to V in the corresponding numbered cavities in Baker's slide.
- Keep the slide in an oven at 55°C.
- Transfer the nematode specimens to solution I and allow for 10 min, then transfer the specimens to solution II and allow for 10 min and continue the same procedure up to solution V.

Composition of Baker's solutions

Composition	I	II	III	IV	V
Glycerine	10	70	82	90	100
Phenol	30	10	5	2.5	0
Lactic acid	30	10	5	2.5	0
Formalin	10	5	3	2.5	0
Distilled water	20	5	5	2.5	0

Mounting

Temporary mounting

a. Water mount

- Place a drop of water in a clear glass slide of dimension 76 x 25 mm.
- Transfer few nematodes from the nematode suspension to the slide.
- Drop a cover slip of 1.9 cm diameter carefully and seal the edges using glyceel/nail polish (cutex) to prevent the evaporation of water.

b. Fixative mount

A drop of fixative is used to mount the nematodes instead of water in the above procedure.

Semipermanent mounting

- Place nematodes in a drop of warm lactophenol in a slide and heat for 3-4 seconds.
- Transfer the nematodes to a drop of dehydrated glycerine.
- Arrange 8 nematodes in 2 rows and arrange similar size 3 glass rods in a triangular position.
- Apply cover slip carefully and drain the excess fluid.
- Seal the edge of cover slip with nail polish and label the slide.

Permanent mounting

Mounts in glycerine can rightly be called 'permanent'; if they are sealed well, they can be permanently stored. They are usually made in Cobb slides. Different materials may be used to support the cover slip, e.g. a paraffin ring or glass fibre.

Requirements

Cobb's slide : Aluminium holder

Square cover slip (25 x 25 mm)

Circular cover slip (18 mm)

Two pieces of cardboard (25 x 25 mm)

Procedure

- ❖ Place a droplet of dehydrated glycerine in the centre of the square cover slip.
- ❖ Transfer the fixed nematode(s) to the middle of the droplet with a pick.
- ❖ Place three glass wool pieces of size slightly larger than the nematode specimens in the droplet at triangle position.
- ❖ Apply a round cover slip with a pair of forceps.
- ❖ Seal the round cover slip with glyceel or nail polish or paraffin wax

- Insert into the Cobb's aluminum slide.
- Place two pieces of cardboard on either side of the cover slip.

Cobb's Aluminum slide

Cobb's Aluminium slide with a hole at the center can be used to mount the nematode. The dimension of the slide is 76 x 25mm with 0.38mm thickness.

Advantages

- The specimens can be viewed from both sides.
- Vertical arrangement of slides makes it easier and safer for long distance transport.
- Lesser risk of breakage of slides.

7

Classification of Plant Parasitic Nematodes Based on Their Feeding Habit

The nematode feeding on plant can be divided into above ground feeders and below ground feeders.

I. Above ground feeders

a) Feeding on flower buds, leaves and bulbs

i) Seed gall nematode : *Anguina tritici*

ii) Leaf and bud nematode : *Aphelenchoides*

iii) Stem and buld nematode : *Ditylenchus*

b) Feeding on tree trunk

i) Red ring nematode : *Bursaphelenchus cocophilus*

ii) Pine wilt nematode : *Bursaphelenchus xylophilus*

According to the mode of parasitism, the nematodes can be divided into

1. Ectoparasitic nematodes,
2. Semi endoparasitic nematodes and
3. Endoparasitic nematodes

II. Below ground feeders

	Endoparasite		Semiendoparasite		Ectoparasite
	Sedentary		Migratory		
i)	Cyst nematode	i)	Lesion nematode	**i)**	Citrus nematode
	Heterodera spp		*Pratylenchus* spp		*Tylenchulus semipenetrans*
	Globodera spp	ii)	Burrowing nematode	ii)	Reniform nematode

ii)	Root-knot nematode		*Radopholus similis*		*Rotylenchulus reniformis*
	Meloidogyne spp	iii)	Rice root nematode		
			Hirschmanniella spp		
	Sedentary		Migratory		
i)	Sheath nematode	i)	Needle nematode	:	*Longidorus* sp.
	Hemicriconemoides spp	ii)	Dagger nematode	:	*Xiphinema* sp.
	Hemicyclophora spp.	iii)	Stubby nematode	:	*Trichodorus* sp.
	Cacopaurus spp	iv)	Pin nematode	:	*Paratylenchus* sp

1. Ectoparasitic nematodes

These nematodes live freely in the soil and move closely or on the root surface, feed intermittently on the epidermis and root hairs near the root tip.

a. *Migratory ectoparasite* : (e.g.) *Criconemoides* spp., *Paratylenchus* spp. and *Trichodorus* spp. These nematodes spend their entire life cycle free in the soil, feeding externally on the host plants, deposit eggs in soil. When the roots are disturbed they detach themselves.

b. *Sedentary ectoparasites* : (e.g.) *Hemicycliophora arenaria* and *Cacopaurus pestis*. In this type of parasitism the attachment of nematode to the root system is permanent but for this, it is similar to the previous one.

2. Semi-endoparasitic nematodes

(e.g.) *Rotylenchulus reniformis* and *Tylenchulus semipenetrans*. The anterior part of the nematode, head and neck being permanently fixed in the cortex and the posterior part extends free into the soil.

3. Endoparasitic nematodes

The entire nematode is found inside the root and the major portion of nematode body found inside the plant tissue.

a. *Migratory endoparasite*: (e.g.) *Hirschmanniella* spp,, *Pratylenchus* spp. and *Radopholus similis*. These nematodes move in the cortial parenchyma of host root. While migrating they feed on cells, multiply and cause necrotic lesions.

b. *Sedentary endoparasite*: (e.g.) *Heterodera* spp. and *Meloidogyne* spp. The second stage juveniles penetrate the root lets and become sedentary throughout the life cycle, inside the root cortex.

8

Nematode Disease Symptoms on Crop Plants

Most of the plant parasitic nematodes affect the root portion of plants except *Anguina* spp., *Aphelenchus* spp., *Aphelenchoides* spp., *Ditylenchus* spp., *Bursaphelenchus cocophilus* and *B. xylophilus*. Nematodes suck the sap of the plants with the help of stylet and causes leaf discolouration, stunted growth, reduced leaf size and fruits, lesions on roots, galls, reduced root system and finally wilting.

Symptoms of nematode diseases can be classified as

I. Symptoms produced by above ground feeding nematodes

II. Symptoms produced by below ground feeding nematodes

I. Symptoms produced by above ground feeding nematodes

1. *Leaf discolouration*: The leaf tip become white in rice due to rice white tip nematode, *Aphelenchoides besseyi*, yellowing of leaves on chrysanthemum due to chrysanthemum foliar nematode, *A. ritzemabosi.*
2. *Dead or devitalised buds*: In case of strawberry plants infected with *A. fragariae*, the nematodes affect the growing point and kill the plants and result in blind plant.
3. *Seed galls* : In wheat, *Anguina tritici* juvenile enter into the flower primordium and develops into a gall. The nemotodes can survive for longer period (even upto 28 years) inside the cockled wheat grain.
4. *Twisting of leaves and stem* : In onion, the basal leaves become twisted when infested with *Ditylenchus dipsaci* and in rice the top leaves become twisted when infested with *D. angustus*.
5. *Crinkled or distorted stem and foliage* : The wheat seed gall nematode, *A. tritici* infests the growing point as a result distortions in stem and leaves takes place.

6. *Necrosis and discolouration* : The red ring disease on coconut is caused by *Bursaphelenchus cocophilus*. Due to the infestation, red coloured circular area appear in the trunk of the infested palm.

7. *Lesions on leaves and stem* : Small yellowish spots are produced on onion stem and leaves due to *D. dipsaci* and the leaf lesions caused by *A. ritzemabosi* on chrysanthemum.

II. Symptoms produced by below ground feeding nematodes

The nematodes infest and feed on the root portion and exhibit symptoms on below ground plant parts as well as on the above ground plants parts and they are classified as

a) Above ground symptoms

b) Below ground symptoms

a. Above ground symptoms

1) *Stunting* : Reduced plant growth and the plants cannot able to withstand adverse conditions. Patches of stunted plants appear in the field. (eg.) in potato due to *Globodera rostochiensis,* in gingelly, due to *Heterodera cajani* and in wheat by *Heterodera avenae*.

2) *Discolouration of foliage* : Patchy yellow appearance in coffee due to *Pratylenchus coffeae* and *G. rostochiensis* infested potato plants show light green foliage. *Tylenchulus semipenetrans* induce fine mottling on the leaves of orange and lemon trees.

3) *Decline and dieback* : In banana, decline and die-back are caused by *Radopholus similis*, spreading decline in cirtus due to *R. citrophilus* and slow decline of cirtus due to *Tylenchulus semipenetrans*. In grapevine slow decline is caused by *Meloidogyne* spp.

4) *Wilting* : Day wilting due to *Meloidogyne* spp. i.e. In hot weather the root-knot infested plants tend to droop or wilt even in the presence of enough moisture in the soil. Severe damage to the root system due to nematode infestation leads to day wilting especially in broad leaved plants like tobacco and brinjal.

b. Below ground symptoms

1. *Root galls or knots* : The characteristic roots galls are produced by root-knot nematode, *Meloidogyne* spp. False root galls are produced by *Nacobbus batatiformis* on sugarbeet and tomato. Small galls are produced

by *Hemicycliophora arenaria* on lemon roots. *Ditylenchus radicicola* causes root galls on wheat and oats. *Xiphinema diversicaudatum* causes galls on rose roots.

2. *Root lesions* : The penetration and movement of nematodes in the root causes typical root lesions e.g. Necrotic lesions induced by *Pratylenchus* spp on crossandra; the burrowing nematode, *Radopholous similis* in banana. Similarly *Pratylenchus coffeae* and *Helicotylenchus multicinctus* cause reddish brown lesion on banana root and corm. The rice root nematode also causes brown lesions on rice root.

3. *Reduced root system* : Due to nematode feeding the root tip growth is arrested and the root produce branches. This may be of various kinds such as coarse root, stubby root and curly tip.

    a. *Coarse root* : *Paratrichodorus* spp. infestation arrest the growth of lateral roots and leads to an open root system with only main roots without lateral roots.

    b. *Stubby roots* : The lateral roots produce excessive rootlets (e.g. *P. christei*)

    c. *Curly tip* : In the injury caused by *Xiphinema* spp. the nematode retards the elongation of roots and causes curling of roots known as 'Fish hook' symptom.

4. *Root proliferation* : Increase in the root growth or excessive branching due to nematode infestation. The infested plant root produces excessive root hair at the point of nematode infestaion. (eg.) *Trichodorus christei, Nacobbus* spp, *Heterodera* spp. *Meloidogyne hapla* and *Pratylenchus* spp.

5. *Root rot* : The nematodes feed on the fleshy structure result in rotting of tissues (e.g.) Yam nematode *Scutellonema bradys* in *Diascorea* spp. and *Ditylenchus destructor* in potato.

6. *Root surface necrosis* : The severe injury caused by *T. semipenetrans* on citrus leads to complete decortication of roots and results in root necrosis.

7. *Cluster of sprouts on tubers* : On the tubers, clusters of short and swollen sprouts are formed due to *D. dipsaci* infestation in many tuber plants.

9

Interaction of Nematodes with Microorganism

Plant parasitic nematodes favour the establishment of secondary pathogens *viz.*, fungi, bacteria, virus etc. The nematodes alter the host in such a way that the host tissue becomes suitable for colonization by the secondary pathogens. Even though the nematodes themselves are capable of causing considerable damage to the crops, their association with other organisms aggravate the disease. The nematodes cause mechanical wound which favours the entry of microorganisms. In some cases, the association of nematode and pathogen breaks the disease resistance in resistant cultivators of crop plants.

Nematode - Fungus Interaction

Nematode - fungus interaction was first observed by Atkinson (1892) in cotton. *Fusarium* wilt was more severe in the presence of *Meloidogyne* spp. Since then the nematode - fungus interations had received considerable attention on important crops like banana, cotton, cowpea, brinjal, tobacco and tomato. Some examples of nematode - fungus interaction are given in the following table.

Crop	Name of the	Nematode	Fungus	Role of disease nematode
Cotton	Damping off	*Meloidogyne incognita acrita*	*Rhizoctonia solani*	Assists
		M.incognita acrita debaryanum	*Pythium* sp.	Assists
	Vascular wilt	*M. incognita acrita F. vasinfectum*	*Fusarium oxysporum*	Assists
		Rotylenchulus reniformis	F. oxysporum f.sp. vasinfectum	Assists
		Belonolaimus gracilis	*F. oxysporum* f.sp. *vasinfectum*	Assists
		B. longicaudatus vasinfectum	F. oxysporum f.sp.	Assists
	Black shank (vascular wilt) nicotianae	*M. incognita acrita*	*Phytophthora parasitica* var.	Assists

Crop	Name of the	Nematode	Fungus	Role of disease nematode
Tobacco	Damping off	*M. incognita acrita*	*P. debaryamum*	Assists
		M. incognita	*Alternaria tenuis*	Assists
	Vascular wilt nicotianae	*M. incognita*	*F. oxysporum* f.sp.	Assists
		M. incognita acrita	*P. parsitica* var *nicotianae*	Assists
Banana	Vascular wilt Essential	*Radopholus similis ubense*	*F. oxysporum* f.sp.	
Tomato	Cortical rot rostochiensis Vascular wilt	*Globodera*	*R. solani*	Assists
		Meloidogyne spp.	*F. oxysporum* f. sp. *lycopersici*	Assits
Potato	Damping off Cortial rot	*Ditylenchus destructor* *G.rostochiensis* *G.rostochiensis*	*P. infestans* *R. solani* Vetricillium dahliae	Assists Assists Assists
Onion	Damping off	*D.dipsaci*	*Botrytis allii*	Assists
Brinjal	Vascular wilt	*P. penetrans*	*V. albo-atrum*	Assists
Pea	Vascular wilt	*Pratylenchus* spp.	*F. oxysporum* f. sp.	Assists
		P. penetrans	pisi f. pisi	Assists
		Hoplolaimus spp.	F. oxyporum f.sp f. pisi	
Soybean	Damping off	*M. javanica*	*R.solani*	Assists
	Vascular wilt	*Heterodera glycines*	*Fusarium* sp.	Assists
Cowpea	Vascular wilt	*M.javanica*	*F. oxysporum* f.sp. *tracheiphylum*	Assists
Lucerne	Vascular wilt	*M. hapla vasinfectum*	*F. oxysporum* f.sp.	Assists
Tulip, Narcissus	Cortical rot	*P. penetrans*	*Cylindrocarpon radicicola*	Assists
Carnation	Vascular wilt	*Meloidogyne* spp.	*F. oxysporum* f.sp. *dianthi*	Assists
Wheat	Stem rot Wheat rot	*Auguina tritici* *H. avenae*	*Dilophospora* *Essential alopecuri* *R. solani*	Assists

Nematode - Bacterium Interactions

Nematode - bacterium interactions are comparatively fewer than the nematode - fungas interactions. Some examples of nematode - bacterial associations are presented in the following table.

Crop	Name of the	Nematode	Bacterium	Role of diseasedisease
Wheat	Tundu	*A. tritici*	*C. clavibacter*	Essential
Tobacco	Vascular wilt	*M. incognita solanacearum*	*Pseudomonas*	Assists
Tomato	Vascular wilt	*M. hapla, M. incognita*	*P. solanacearum*	Assists
	Vascular wilt	*Helicotylenchus nannus*	*P. solanacearum*	Assists
	Canker	*M. incognita*	*C. michiganensis var michiganensis*	Assists
Potato	Vascular wilt	*Meloidogyne* spp.	*P. solanacearum*	Assists
Lucerne	Crown buds (vasucular wilt)	*D. dipsaci*	*C. insidiosum*	Essential &Assists
Raspberry	Crown gall	*M. halpa*	*Agrobacterium tumefasciens*	Assists
Strawberry	Cauliflower disease	*Aphelenchodies ritzemobosi*	*C. fascians*	Essential
Peach	Crown gall	*M. javanica*	*A. tumefasciens*	Assists
Peach, Plum	Canker	*Criconemella xenoplex*	*P. syringae*	Assists
Begonia	Leaf spot	*A. fragariae*	*Xanthomonas begoniae*	Assists
Carnation	Root (Vascular wilt)	*Meloidogyne* spp. *H. dihystera*	*P. caryophylli*	Assists
Rose	Hairy root	*P. vulnus*	*A. rhizogenes*	Assists
Gladiolus	Scab	*M. javanica*	*P. marginata*	Assists

Nematode - Virus Interaction

In nematode virus complex, nematode serves as a vector. Numerous virus-nematode complexes have been identified after the pioneer work by Hewit, Raski and Goheen (1958) who found that *Xiphinema index* was the vector of grapevine fan leaf virus. *Xiphinema* spp., *Longidorus* spp. and *Paralongidorus* spp. transmit the ring spot viruses which are called "NEPO" derived from Nematode transmitted polyhedral shaped particles. *Trichodorus* spp. and *Paratrichodorus* spp. transmit the rattle viruses and called "NETU" derived from Nematode tranmitted tubular shaped particles. All these nematodes have modified bottle shaped oesophagus with glands connected by short ducts directly to the lumen of the oesophagus. This actually helps in the transmission of viruses which is different in other genera of nematodes. Certain examples of the viral diseases and the nematode vectors are given in the following table.

Viruses	**Nematode**
NEPO- Viruses	
Arabis mosaic	*Xiphinema diversicaudatum*
	X. paraelongatum
Arabis mosaic, Grapevine fan leaf	*X. index*
Arabis mosaic, Grapevine	*X. index*
Yellow mosaic	
Strawberry latent ring spot	*X. diversicaudatum*
Tobacco ring spot,	*X. americanum*
Tobacco ring spot, Peach Yellow bud mosaic	*X. americanum*
Cowpea mosaic	*X. basiri*
Arabis mosaic, Raspberry ring spot,	*Paralongidorus maximus*
Strawberry latent ring spot	
Raspberry ring spot - Scottish strain	*Longidorus elongaatus*
Raspberry ring spot - English strain	*L. macrosoma*
Tomato black ring, Beet ring spot	*L. elongatus*
Tomato black ring, Lettuce ring spot	*L. attenuatus*
NETU - Viruses	
Tobacco	*Paratrichodorus pachydermus, P. allius, P. nanus, P. porosus, P. teres Trichodorus christei T. primitivus, T. cylindricus T. hooperi, T. minor, T. similis*
Pea early browning	*P. anemones, P. pachydermus P. teres, T. viruliferus*

Nematodes acquire and transmit the virus by feeding, which requires as little as one day. Once acquired, the virus persists for longer period in the nematode body than *in vitro*. For example, the grapevine fan leaf virus will exist for as many as 60 days in *X. index*. Two types of mechanisms are observed in virus transmission (i) retention through close biological association between virus and vector as in *Xiphinema*; (ii) retention of virus mechanically as in *Longidorus*. Virus is retained in the inner surface of the guiding sheath of *Longidorous*, cuticle lining of the lumen of oesophagus in *Trichodorus* and *Paratrichodrous*, cuticle lining of stylet extension and oesophagus in *Xiphinema*. The virus particles are released into plant cell with the help of oesophagus.

10

Nematode Pests of Field Crops

Rice

Plant parasitic nematodes cause serious damage to rice crop. Thirty two species belonging to 13 genera were observed in association with the crop. Among them few are considered to be important. They are the rice white - tip nematode (*Aphelenchoides besseyi*), rice stem nematode (*Ditylenchus angustus*), rice root nematode (*Hirschmanniella oryzae*), root-knot nematode (*Meloidogyne graminicola*) and the cyst nematode (*Heterodera oryzicola*).

The white-tip nematode *(Aphelenchoides besseyi)*

The yield loss due to the white-tip nematode is estimated to be as much as 17.4 to 54.1 per cent. The nematode is distributed in India, Bangladesh, Sri Lanka, Japan, Indonesia, Taiwan, Former USSR, Italy, Cuba and Madagascar.

Symptoms

Infected seeds emerge late in seed beds and produce small seedlings. The upper 2 to 5 cm leaf tip turn white or pale yellow in the tillering stage and then turn brown. Flag leaves are characteristically shortened and twisted at their apical portions. Panicles are shorter and spilelets are reduced which inturn produce deformed kernels. The infested spiklet show numerous nematodes while examining under a microscope (Plate 1). The nematode delays the maturity of panicles and secondary panicles arise from lower nodes.

Life cycle

The nematode is carried beneath the hull of the kernel in quiescent, immature pre-adult stage. In this quiescent stage the nematode can remain dormant for 2 years. When such infested seeds are sown, the nematode revive and move to the growing points of the leaf and stem and feed ectoparasitically. The eggs are deposited in the leaf axis or in panicles and many generations occur in one season. Reproduction follows plant growth and the nematodes move upward along with the development of leaf. Movement of nematodes are mostly due to the presence of thin film of moisture due to rain or dew or high humidity.

Many nematodes enter into the panicles and some nematodes found inside the hull. Normally 5 to 6 nematodes are found in each seed. The life cycle takes 8 days at 23°C and 10 days at 21°C.

Host range

The nematode also infests *Setaria italica, S. viridis, Panicum sanguinale* and *Cyperus iria.* Apart from this strawberry, tuberose, chrysanthemum, *Boehmeria nivea, Ficus elastica* and *Pennisetum typhoides* are also reported to be the hosts for the nematode.

Spread and survival

The spread is mainly by infested seeds. The nematode is also carried along with irrigation water to nearby fields. Second stage juveniles remain in quiescent stage outside or inside the husk and can survive for 3 years in this stage but die in 4 months on grain left in the field and they cannot survive in the soil. Rice seedlings growing from shed grain may allow the nematodes to survive from one season to the next.

Management

1. Use of certified seeds can eliminate the nematode.
2. Hot water treatment of seeds at 55°C for 15 minutes prior to sowing or seed disinfestation by sun drying for 12 hours between 9 am and 3 pm for 2 days.
3. Burning of stubbles after harvest for preventing perpetuation of the nematode in field through dormant nematodes.
4. Spraying monocrotophos 36 EC at 1000 ml/ha at the boot-leaf stage in 500 litres of water.

The rice stem nematode *(Ditylenchus angustus)*

The rice stem nematode was first reported by Butler (1913) from rice producing region, north of the Bay of Bengal and east of the Ganges river (Bangladesh). The nematode can cause yield reduction from 20 to 50 per cent.

Geographical distribution

The rice stem nematode has been reported to occur in Bangaladesh, India, Burma, Malaya, Thailand, Philippines and Madagascar.

Symptoms

The nematode causes **'ufra'** disease in rice. Initial chlorosis or streaks appear on the leaves. There are 2 distinct types of symptoms, one is the **'swollen ufra'** and another called **'ripe ufra'.** In the first type, the panicle remains enclosed within the leaf sheath and branching occurs in the infested portions. In ripe ufra the panicle emerge and produces normal grain only near the tip. The panicle turns dark brown and lower flowers in the panicle remains unfertilized.

Life cycle

Cottony like masses **(nematode wool)** of pre adult fourth stage juveniles are formed in the infested plants. During humid periods they become active, move to the upper part of the plant and invade the growing point. The nematode feed ectoparasitically on the epidermal cells of the young seed head, the peduncle and the part of stem just above the upper nodes. Rolling of young leaves are also noticed. Developing heads are found to contain large number of nematodes from egg stage to adult stage.

Spread and survival

Cottony masses of nematodes are seen in anabiosis state in the plant parts at the end of growing season. Some of the nematodes remain on the stubbles even after harvest. When rainy season starts, the cottony masses of nematodes in anabiosis state revive and infect the new crop. The nematode also spreads through irrigation water. The nematode can survive desiccation for more than 15 months as cottony masses.

Management

Crop rotation with jute, avoiding water-logged condition by providing proper drainage, destruction of stubbles after harvest and using nematode free seeds are the cultural methods for the management of the nematode.

Spraying Diazinon 100 ppm on the soil in the rice crop controls the nematodes within 72 hours. 'Khao Tah Oo' a resistant rice variety to blast disease is also resistant to the rice stem nematode.

The rice-root nematode *(Hirschmanniella oryzae)*

The rice root nematode is also associated with the **'mentek'** disease of rice, where the plant root show severe infestation which leads to very poor growth. The rice root nematode is wide spread throughout the rice growing regions of India. This nematode can cause a yield loss from 10 to 30 per cent depending upon the infestation load.

Geographical distribution

The nematode is found to occur in Indonesia, Malaysia, India, Thailand, Japan, Philippines, Nigeria, Taiwan, Sri Lanka and USA.

Symptoms

The above ground symptoms are reddish brown discolouration of leaves and stuned growth of plants in patches. The infested plant root show discolouration of roots and rotting. The nematode is a migratory endoparasite and feeds on the cortical cells.

Life cycle

Both male and female nematodes invade the roots through the epidermis. The opening caused by the entrance of one individual is used by other nematodes resulting in concentration of nematodes in the infested part. The nematode enter near the root tip and subsequently invade the cortical cells. The life cycle is completed in 30 days.

Survival

Weeds like *Echinochloa, Cyperus, Monochloria* and *Marsilia* are found to harbour the nematodes. After harvest the left out rice stubbles harbour enourmous nematodes which can infest the next crop.

Management

Summer ploughing and removal and destruction of stubbles reduce the infestation for the next season crop.

Carbofuran 3G @ 170 g/cent of nursery reduces the infestation in young seedlings.

The root-knot nematode (*Meloidogyne graminicola*)

M. graminicola is a problem in upland rice and causes yield loss upto 50 per cent. *M. incognita* and *M. javanica* are also found to infest rice roots and cause severe root galls.

Geographical distribution

The nematode infestation is reported from USA, Thailand, Bangladesh, India and Laos. In India, *M. graminicola, M. javanica* and *M. incognita* are often observed in Assam, Orissa, Madhya Pradesh, West Bengal, Tiripura, Kerala and some parts of Tamil Nadu.

Symptoms

Leaves of affected plants become discoloured from 10 to 12 days after infestation by the second stage juveniles. Leaves change to bronze colour from marigins towards the midrib. Severe infestation results in stunted growth. The infested plant root shows typical galls like beads or clubs around the region where the nematode fix the feeding site (Plate 2). Growth of the root is retarded and profuse development of side roots takes place.

Life cycle

The life cycle is completed in 26 to 51 days depending upon the climatic condition. The J_2 enter the roots at the zone of elongation and migrate intercellularly. At feeding site giant cells are formed which inturn affect the xylem vessels. The female nematode on maturity lays 200 - 300 eggs in gelatinous matrix which protrude out of the root.

Management

Amending soil with decaffeinated tea waste and water hyacinth compost reduces the nematode infestation.

Flooding the soil and destruction of alternate weed hosts reduces the population in soil.

Crop rotation with french bean and jute reduces nematode infestation

Rice varieties like TKM 6, Patna 6, Dumai, Ch 47 and Hamsa are resistant to the nematode.

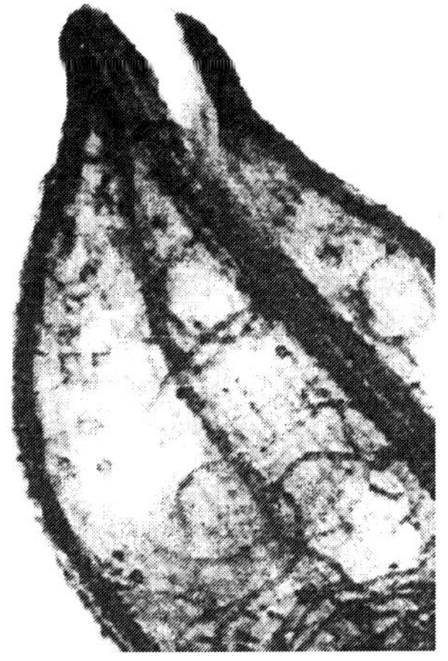

Plate 1. Rice white tip nematode infested spikelet

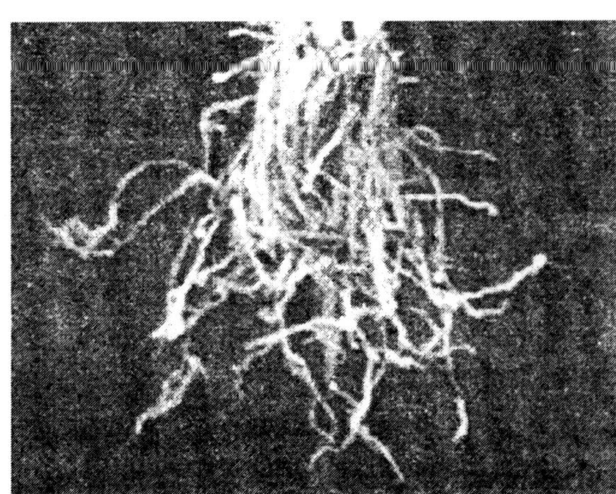

Plate 2. Rice root showing severe root-galls due to root-knot nematode infestation

Wheat

India ranks fourth among the wheat growing countries of the world. Wheat is grown in states like Utter Pradesh, Punjab, Madhya Pradesh, Rajasthan, Bihar and Haryana.

The important nematodes that cause damage to wheat are the cereal cyst nematode and seed gall nematode.

The cereal cyst nematode (*Heterodera avenae*)

Kuhn (1874) first reported the cereal cyst nematode in Germany. Later, Prasad *et al.* (1959) reported the nematode on wheat in India. This nematode causes **'molya'** disease in wheat and barley.

Geographical distribution

The nematode occurs in countries like Germany, Sweden, Denmark, Netherlands, Norway, Japan, Australia, Canada, Israel, South Africa, North Africa and India. In India, the nematode occurs in Rajasthan, Haryana, Punjab, Himachal Pradesh and Jammu & Kashmir.

Symptoms

The nematode infested field shows a patchy appearance. Continuous cropping of wheat and barley leads to multiplication of the nematode and the whole field start showing the symptoms. The damage is severe during the dry season. The infested plants show stunted growth and chlorosis. The affected plant leaves have stiff, thin and narrow leaf blades. Tillering is very much reduced. Premature flowering is observed in infested plants and such plants have only few grains.

Life cycle

Dark brown coloured lemon shaped cysts can be recovered from the infested field in large numbers. The cysts can also be recovered from infested root and soil. Each cyst may contain 200-300 eggs and juveniles. These eggs and juveniles remain dormant until the next host crop (wheat or barley) is available. When the cooler season starts, the infective second stage juveniles start emerging from the cysts. After emergence, the J_2 penetrate the root and remain as sedentary endoparasite. The J_2 develop in 25-30 days and become adult. Lemon shaped white females can be seen protruding out of the roots in about 35 days after penetration.

The white females die and the body wall hardens due to quinone tanning and can be seen as brown coloured cysts. These cysts are tough and leathery and can withstand adverse conditions. These cysts enclosing eggs, fall in the soil and serve as a source of inoculum for the next crop. The nematode completes its life cycle within 9 to 14 weeks of juveniles invasion.

Host range

Wheat, barley, oats, rye and maize are some of the host plants for the nematode.

Spread and survival

The cereal cyst nematode spread through implements, soil adhering the labour feet and also along with irrigation water.

The cyst remains viable in the soil for several years without the host plant.

Management

Non-host crops like carrot, fenugreek, onion, mustard and gram can be included in the crop rotation.

Carbofuran 3G or aldicarb 10G can be applied @ 1.5 kg. a.i/ha.

Resistant varieties can be grown. Hannchen, Chevalier Primus and Schwannhals are some of the barley varieties resistant to *H. avenae.*

The Wheat seed-gall nematode (*Anguina tritici*)

Needham (1743) first reported the seed gall nematode. It was the first plant parasitic nematode identified and still it is one of the most important plant parasitic nematode of wheat in India. The nematode causes **'ear-cockle'** disease in wheat. The nematode in association with bacterium, *Corynebacterium clavibacter* causes **'tundu'** disease in wheat.

Geographical distribution

The nematode is reported to occur in countries like England, Sweden, Netherlands, France, Germany, Austria, Hungary, Switzerland, Italy, Egypt, Israel, Syria, Pakistan, China, Australia, New Zealand, USA and Brazil. In India, the seed gall nematode is a serious problem in all wheat growing northern states.

Symptoms

Infested seedlings show slight enlargement of the basal part of the stem. Leaves emerging from infected plants are twisted, crinkled and often folded with their tips held near the growing point. Severely infested seedlings are stunted and even die prematurely. Profuse tillering can be observed in infested plants. The infested plant ears are usually shorter. Glumes are spread farther apart by the galls, which replace the kernels. Seed galls are smaller, shorter and dark in colour compared to healthy grains.

The 'tundu' disease is characterised by the production of a light yellow slime on the leaf surfaces of young plants and also on the abortive ears. The yellow slime in some cases can be seen trickling down the tissues in humid weather and later on becomes hard, brittle and brown on drying. Emerging spike is narrower and shorter, with the grains partially or completely replaced by the bacterial mass and in some cases fails to emerge out of the boot leaf. The stalk is distorted when the ear shows bacterial symptoms.

Life cycle

The seed galls fall in the field during harvest and break down in the soil to release the second stage juveniles. Each seed gall may contain 3000 to 12,000 J_2 depending upon the size of the gall. The J_2 invade the seedling and move to the aerial part and feed ecto-parasitically in the growing point and leaf sheath. During embryonic flower formation, the nematode invade them and shift from ectoparasitic to endoparasitic life. The nematodes develop into adult in the developing seed, which becomes a gall. Mating occurs and the females lay thousands of eggs. The adult die and the eggs hatch. The juveniles moult once in the gall to have J_2 in seed gall. The J_2 in seed galls remain viable for several years.

Host range

Wheat, rye and *Triticum dicoccum* are susceptible to the seed gall nematode. Oats and barley are immune to the nematode.

Spread and survival

The main spread of the nematode is through the seed galls along with the seed grains. The J_2 can remain viable for many years in dried seed galls. Contamination of grains with galls beyond 5 per cent by weight spoil the colour, texture, odour and taste of chapatis.

Management

Dry cleaning of seeds or Brine flotation

Dry cleaning methods like sieving and winnowing eliminates the galled seeds from healthy seeds. Seed floatation with 20 per cent brine solution also helps to eliminate the galled seeds.

Hot water treatment

The seeds are presoaked in cold water for 4 to 6 hours and then treated in hot water (54°C) for 10 minutes. This treatment kills the nematode in the seed gall.

Seed certification

Seed supplying agencies, both the private and public sectors have an important role in preventing the recurrence and spread of the nematode by distributing nematode free certified seeds.

Crop rotation

Growing non host crops for one or two years eliminates the nematode.

Resistant varieties

'Kenred-a-hard' a winter wheat is resistant to the nematode.

Rogueing

In the field, the infested plants can be detected, removed and destroyed.

Nematode Pest on Pulses

Pulse crops *viz.,* red gram, black gram, green gram, Bengal gram and soybean are rich in protein. The pulses play a vital role in food production. Many pest and diseases are limiting factor in pulse production. Nematode also cause serious damage in pulse crop

Red gram

Red gram, *Cajanus cajan(L.)* is an annual or biennial or perennial crop. The nematode is commonly associated with the crop as cyst nematode, *Heterodera cajani,* root knot nematode *Meloidogyne* spp. and reniform nematode *Rotylenchulus reniformis.* Red gram cyst nematode *Heterodera. cajani*

Symptoms

The infested plants show yellowing and stunting of plants in patches. When closely observed small internodes and leaves can be seen.

Disease complex

The nematode have an association with the wilt pathogen *Fusarium udum* and increase the severity of the disease.

Management

Crop rotation with cereal crops is recommended. Application of carbofuran 3G @ 1 kg ai/ha on 15 days after sowing the seeds

Blackgram

Black gram, *Phaseolus mungo (L)* is cultivated in many tropical and subtropical countries. The crop considered to be native of India. It is also grown in Bangladesh, Pakistan, Burma and Srilanka. It is an annual herbaceous plant. The nematodes commonly associated with crop are cyst nematode, (*Heterodera. cajani*), reniform nematode (*Rotylenchulus reniformis*), root knot nematode (*M.incognita*) and stunt nematode (*Tylenchorhynchous mashoodi*)

Symptoms of damage

The nematode infestation cause stunting and chlorosis in the crop in patches. The root knot nematode cause root galls which inturn suppress the root nodulation on severe infestation reduction yield observed impairing the grain formation and pod setting.

Management

Crop rotation with rice, seed treatment with neem cake, in field application of neem cake @1t/ha. Seed treatment with *Trichoderma viridae* @ 4g/kg of seed and in field application *Trichoderma viridae* @2. Kg/ha.

Application of carbofuran 3G @ 1.0kg /a.i/ha

Greengram

Mungo or green gram, *Vigna radiata* L. is native of India and is being cultivated from even prehistoric times. In India the crop is cultivated throughout the plains. It is an erect and semi-erect herbaceous annual with a tendency for twining in the upper branches.

Root-knot nematode and reniform nematodes are after associated with the crop

Symptoms of damage

The nematode infestation cause stunting and chlorosis in patches. The root knot nematode cause root galls which in turn suppress the root nodulation in severe infestation reduction yield observed impairing the grain formation and pod setting.

Management

Crop rotation with rice, seed treatment with neem cake, in field application of neem cake @1t/ha. Seed treatment with *Trichoderma viridae* @ 4g/kg of seed and in field application *Trichoderma viridae* @2. Kg/ha.

Application of carbofuran 3G @ 1.0kg /a.i/ha

Chick Pea or Bengal gram

Chick pea, (*Cicer arietinum* L.) is an important pulse crop. It is grown as a cold weather crop throughout India.

The nematodes associated with the crop are root knot nematode, lesion nematode and reniform nematode. The root knot nematodes often associated with the crop and cause root galls

Symptoms of damage

The nematode infestation cause stunting and chlorosis in the crop in patches. The root knot nematode cause root galls which in turn suppress the root nodulation in severe infestation reduction yield observed impairing the grain formation and pod setting.

Management

Crop rotation with rice, seed treatment with neem cake, in field application of neem cake @1t/ha. Seed treatment with *Trichoderma viridae* @ 4g/kg of seed and in field application *Trichoderma viridae* @2. Kg/ha.

Application of carbofuran 3G @ 1.0kg /a.i/ha

Nematode pests on cotton

In cotton two species are grown popularly *Gossypium hirsutum* and *Gossypium barbadense, Gossypium hirsutum* is a small annual sub shrub, 1.5 meters tall, stem usually green or brown, leaves and twigs from globrous to densely hairy. *Gossypium barbadense* is a perennial shrub or annual sub – shrub one to three meters tall. Cotton is grown across a variety of climates and soil types. It is a long duration crop and maintained even 5 to 6 months.

Plant parasitic nematodes are associated with the crop and cause yield loss. The nematodes commonly associated with the crops are reniform nematode *Rotylenchulus reniformis,* lance nematode *Hoplolaimus galeatus,* sting nematode *Belonolaimus longicandatus, Longidorus , Xiphinema* and root knot nematode *Meloidogyne* spp.

Disease complexes

The rhizosphere soil is a niche for many microorganisms *viz,* fungi, bacteria, virus, etc. The disease complexes involving root knot nematode and reniform nematode with fungal pathogens are common. The very common interaction is between root knot nematode with vascular wilt pathogen *Fusarium oxysporum f.sp.vesin.*

Reniform nematode

In reniform nematode more than 10 species are associated with the crop *Rotylenchulus reniformis* and Rotylenchus parvus are important which cause damage to the crop *Rotylenchulus reniformis* is widely distributed in tropical regions of India.

1. Nematode	:	Reniform nematode
2. Systematic position		
Phylum	:	Nematoda
Class	:	Secernentea
Order	:	Tylenchida
Suborder	:	Tylenchina
Super family	:	Tylenchoidea
Family	:	Hoplolaimidae
Sub-family	:	Rotylenchulinae
Genus	:	*Rotylenchulus*
Species	:	*R. reniformis*
3. Major hosts	:	Cotton, cowpea, castor, papaya and vegetables
4. Type of parasitism	:	Semiendoparasite

5. Morphology

Body	:	Small, 0.20 to 0.50 mm.
Head	:	Rounded to conoid, medium sclerotization.
Stylet	:	Small in juvenile and male; well developed in immature and mature females.
Oesophagus	:	Median bulb distinct with valves in immature female
Female	:	Swollen to kidney shaped with irregular anterior part; vulva - prominent in the posterior end (58–72%) of immature and mature females; ovary - didelphic, amphidelphic with a double flexture; tail – conoid to round terminus.
Male	:	Vermiform; stylet and oesophagus reduced, weak median bulb; tail – curved, pointed, bursa absent.
Juvenile	:	Resembling immature female but shorter, lacking vulva and genital tracts.

Biology

Reniform nematode is sedentary semiendoparasite on roots. **The pre-adult**

female is infective stage. Vermiform females insert their anterior most region of the body into the root and start swelling, becoming kidney shaped. Gelatinous matrix is secreted by the female around the body in which eggs are deposited. Second stage juveniles undergo three moults in the soil. Third and fourth stage juveniles do not shed the old cuticle. The nematode can feed upon cortical, pericycle, endodermis and phloem cells and results in the formation of syncytium due to hypertrophy and hyperplasia of the cells.

Life cycle

- The species is bisexual and reproduction is by amphimixis.
- The species has an unusual life cycle. Although a newly hatched second stage larva have well developed stylet, they do not feed. They soon undergo three moults in the soil to become young females and adult males. Third and fourth stage juveniles do not shed the old cuticle. The **pre-adult females are the infective stages**.
- The adult female is an obligate, sedentary, semi endoparasite of roots and reniform / kidney shaped while the males are non – parasitic.
- Vermiform females insert their anterior most region of the body into the root and start swelling, becoming kidney shaped.
- Eggs are deposited in a gelatinous matrix outside the root tissue. When these eggs are placed in water they promptly begin to hatch.
- The life cycle is completed in about 25 days provided the young females have found the host immediately.
- The nematode as a semiendoparasite of sedentary nature induces a specialized nurse cell systems for continuous food supply. The system involves wall expansion of several cells at the feeding site, partial wall dissolution, fusion of neighboring cell protoplasts and finally establishment of a multinucleate **syncytium**. These syncytia are mostly confined to the pericycle. Other pericycle cells are metabolically stimulated but they remain discrete and uninucleate.
- The young infective females destroy the exterior cortical cells of roots and the damage increase when the nematode moves towards the phloem.

Symptoms of nematode

Stunting, Chlorosis, incipient wilting, unthrifty appearance profuse root proliferation and galls are produced in root knot nematode infestation.

Management

Growing resistant varieties (Auburn 623) crop rotation with cowpea and groundnut. Biological control with VAM, *Pasteuria penetrans* and *Pseudomonas flourescens*. Application of carbofuran 3G @ 1kg ai/ha at 25 days after sowing cotton seeds. Summer ploughing helps to reduce the nematode infestation in soil.

Nematode pests in oil seed crops

Groundnut or Peanut

Groundnut (*Arachis hypogaea* L.) is native of Brazil of South America. It is an annual legume and low growing. The nodules are found both on tap root and the lateral root. There are two types (bunchy and spreading type). Peanut is a hardy plant which withstands varying environmental conditions. It grows well in well drained sandyloam soil. Groundnut pods are produced on pegs below the ground and hence vulnerable to plant parasitic nematodes found in the rhizosphere.

Nematodes in groundnut

Root knot nematode (*Meloidogne spp*), Lesion nematode (*Pratylenchus brachyurus*), Ring nematode (*Criconemella ornata*), Sting nematode (*Belonolaimus longicaudatus*), peanut pod nematode (*Ditylenchus africanus*) and stunt nematode (*Tlenchorhynchus brevilineatus*).

Root knot nematode

The species *Meloidogne arenaria*, *Meloidogne javanica* are important nematode pests of groundnut. The nematode penetrates root, pegs and pods. The infested plant show stunting and yellowing in patches. The injury to pods reduces the quality of nuts. Pod rotting is also associated with severe infestation. The nematode also increase the severity of mold caused by *Sclerotium rolfsii* and other soil borne fungal pathogens. The nematode cause serious problem in North America, India, China, Africa and Egypt.

Symptoms of damage

Adult female can be observed in roots, pegs and in pods. The females are pearly white and have pointed neck and head is visible. Eggs are attached to the posterior region of the adult female. Eggmass appear as dirt brownish on the surface of the root galls. Infested plants show yellowing and rust appearance. Galls can be seen in pods and pegs.

Lesion nematode

The lesion nematode is a migratory endoparasite. All the stages are infective. The nematode produce dark coloured necrotic lesions in matured shells. Chlorosis and stunting of plants observed in patches.

Stunt nematode

The stunt nematode *Tylenchorhynchus brevilineatus* observed for the first time in Andhra Pradesh state during 1976 in kalahasti region. Since appeared in kalahasti region.Since appeared in kalahasti region the disease is named as "kalahasti region. The disease is characterized by reduction in pod size and brownish black discolouration of pods. At the site of nematode infestation proliferation of cells takes place hence the margins of lesion have an elevated appearance. Peg ling are very much reduced. In severe infestation the pods are discoloured. The kalahasti disease appear in patches.

Kalahasti malady- *Tylenchorhynchus brevilineatus*

The most important nematode disease of groundnut, which occurs severely on pods. The stunt nematode, *Tylenchorhynchus brevilineatus* has been found to be associated with the Kalahasti malady of groundnut. The nematode may reduce the yield of groundnut by 20-60%.

Distribution: The stunt nematode, *T. brevilineatus* was first observed during 1976 at Kalahasti region of Andhra Pradesh, India. The occurrence of stunt nematode on groundnut has also been reported from Tamil Nadu.

Symptoms

- *T. brevilineatus* induces the disease "Kalahasti malady", which is characterized by reduction in pod size, brownish discoloration of the pod surface and appearance of small brownish yellow lesions on pegs and developing pods.
- The margins of lesions become slightly elevated because of cellular proliferation around the site of nematode infection.
- The nematode infested pod stalks were greatly reduced.
- The surfaces of heavily infested pods become completely discolored.

- The nematode does not affect the seeds within the pods. Affected pods become small, shriveled and show ugly external appearance called "Shutti kaya" in Telugu.
- Plant roots also parasitized but discoloration is less severe than on pods.
- The high inoculum levels resulted in symptoms like brownish to black necrotic lesions on root surface, pod stalks, pod surface and reduction in pod size.
- Plants became stunted with dark green foliage and necrotic lesions could be seen on pod surface (Vemana *et al.*, 1999).
- The disease is generally distributed in patches within fields and more severe in sandy soils.

Management

Crop rotation with non host crops like field corn and other cereal. Summer ploughing and exposing the soil to sunlight reduce soil infestation.

Application of carbofuran 3G @ 1kg ai/ha in 25 days after sowing the seeds.

Nematode pests on Tobacco

Tobacco (*Nicotina tabacum L.*) is widely grown commercial crop in the world. The crop is grown in china, USA, Brazil, Turkey, Greece, Italy and India. In India the crop is said to be introduced by portughese in the seventeeth century. The best quality of tobacco is from the individual leaves as they mature. Curing is required by drying process by which the leaves loose moisture and become tough and reddish brown.

Root knot nematode (*Meloidogyne spp*) is the important nematode which causes considerable damage to the crop. The damage by the nematode is very high in sandy loam soil due to condusive abiotic factors especially the aeration. The nematode produces numerous galls. The infested plants show stunted growth with nutrient deficiency symptom. Boron deficiencies also associated with the nematode infestation. In case of severe infestation premature wilting and stunting observed in patches. Day wilt symptoms also appear in the afternoon of hot days, despite the presence of adequate soil moisture. In Tamilnadu state the crop is grown in vedachandur, kodiakarai, vedharanyam and ottanchatiram villages. In all the tobacco cultivated areas the root knot nematode *Meloidogyne incognita* is the serious menace.

Apart from the root knot nematode the lesion nematode *Pratylenchus spp* is also observed. The nematode is a migratory endoparasite and cause lesions in the root. Initially lesions appear as discrete, elliptical, water soaked area just behind the root tip subsequently the lesions become brown to black colour. On severe infestation the lesion coalesce to grindle the roots.

Both root-knot and lesion nematodes have association with tobacco black shank, fungus *Phytophthora parasitica var nocotiana,* Fusarium wilt caused by *Fusarium oxysporum f. sp nicotinae* and bacterial wilt caused by *Pseudomonas solanacearum.*

Management

Crop rotation with non host crops.

Summer ploughing and exposing field to sunlight

Robbing (burning plant residues) is also practiced is some regions to reduce the soil infestation after the harvest of leaves.

Application of Farmyard manure and neem cake is also found to reduce the nematode infestation by way of host plant nutrition and encouraging nematode antagonistic organisms and release of toxic gases and organic acids

11

Nematode Pests of Fruit Crops

Citrus (*Citrus* spp.)

Citrus is an important fruit crop and ranks third in area which is followed by mango and banana. They are grown in 105,396 hectares in India. Among the oranges, mandarin oranges, limes and sweet oranges are very popular while lemons, grape fruits, pummelos, sour and bitter oranges are of minor importance. The *Citrus* spp. are grown in larger extent in the states of Maharashtra, Karnataka, Kerala, Tamil Nadu, Andhra Pradesh, Punjab, Haryana, Rajasthan, Assam, Orissa and Bihar.

Nematode menace in citrus gardens are very much realised. In 1912 the citrus nematode, *Tylenchulus semipenetrans* was reported from California and found to cause '**slow decline**' disease. More than 30 genera of plant parasitic nematodes are associated with the *Citrus* spp. Among them, *Tylenchulus semipenetrans*, *Radopholus citrophilus, Meloidogyne* spp. *Pratylenchus* spp. *Xiphinema* spp. and *Hoplolaimus* spp. are often associated with the crop.

The citrus nematode (*Tylenchulus semipenetrans*)

The citrus nematode, *T.semipenetrans* is a very important nematode parasite in citrus. It is a semi-endoparasite found to insert its head and neck inside the root and the remaining posterior portions of the body outside the root (Plate 4A&B). This nematode causes slow decline and considered to be one of the factors responsible for die-back disease of citrus trees in India. The annual reduction in world citrus crop yield due to this nematode is estimated to be 8.7 to 12.2 per cent.

Geographical distribution

The citrus nematode is distributed in all citrus growing areas in the world. In India, it has been reported from Uttar Pradesh, Delhi, Punjab, Rajasthan, Maharashtra, West Bengal, Assam, Himachal Pradesh, Sikkim, Orissa, Haryana, Bihar, Karnataka, TamilNadu and Andhra Pradesh.

Symptoms

Nematode infestation in citrus results in reduction of tree growth and vigour. Yellowing and shedding of leaves are often noticed. The symptoms are mostly produced in the uppermost branches of the tree. If the nematode is not controlled, the symptoms will spread to lower part of the tree (Plate 3). The infected tree produces small fruits. If the infected tree roots are examined by gentle washing and boiling the roots in acid fuschin lactophenol, the adult females can be seen through stereoscopic microscope as semiendoparasite. In heavily infested roots, the cortex separates readily from the vascular stele.

Life cycle

Van Gundy (1958) studied the life cycle. Eggs hatch in 12 to 14 days at about 24^{0}C and sex differentiation is possible at the second stage juveniles. The second stage male juveniles develop into adult within 7 days without feeding. The second stage female juveniles require 14 days to locate the root, feed on the epidermal cells and moult. The life cycle from egg to egg requires 6 to 8 weeks.

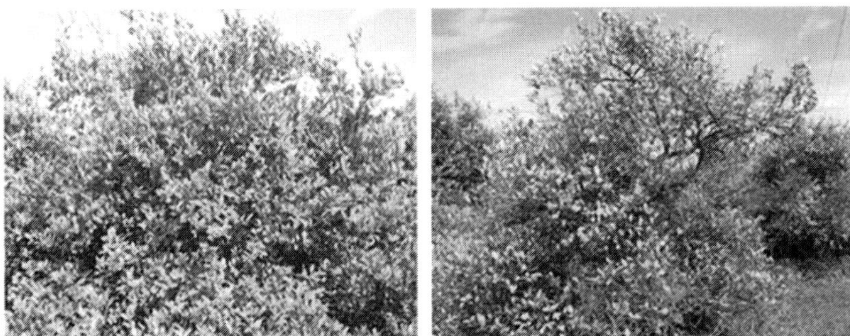

Plate 3: Citrus tree infested with *T. semipenetrans*

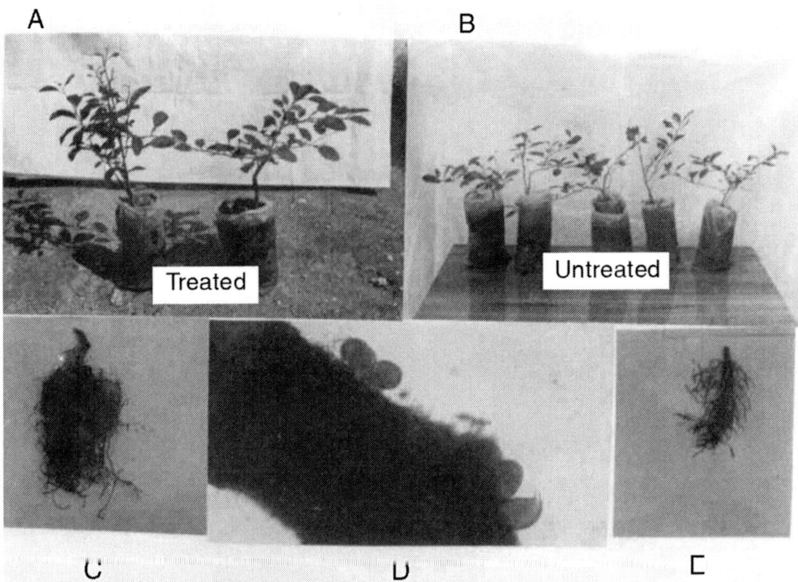

Plate 4: **A.** Healthy seedling **B.** Infested seedling **C.** Healthy seedling root **D.** Affected root **E.** Females attached to citrus root

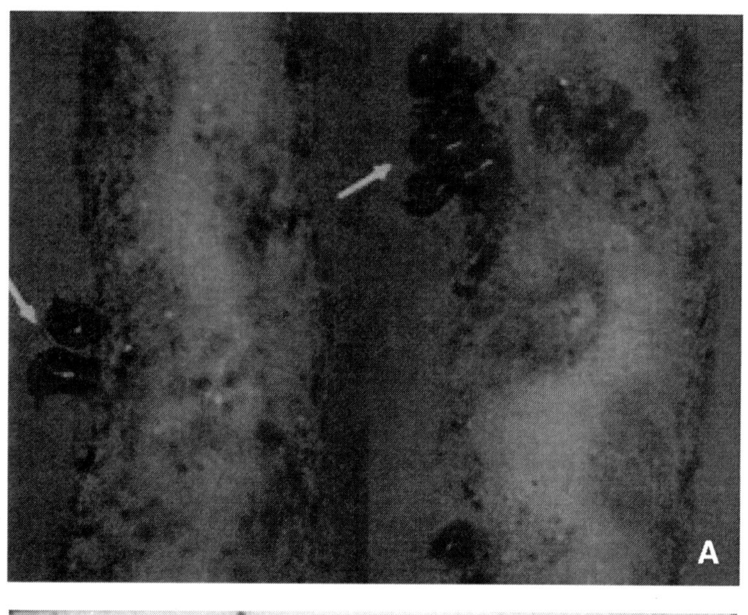

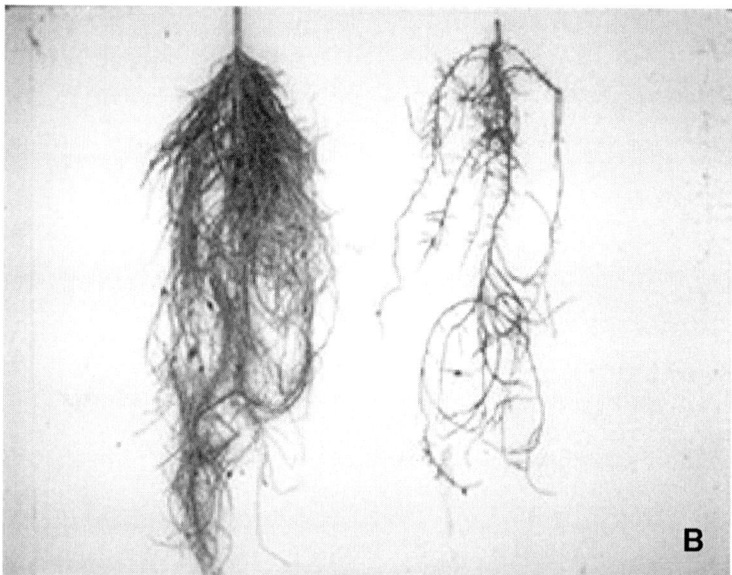

Plate 4A: A. Females attached to roots **B.** Healthy and infested seedling roots

Host parasitic relationship

The second stage juveniles which are 4 to 5 weeks old penetrate the roots and feed on them. The young females penetrate deeper and become established at a depth of several cortical cells. A feeding site is developed around the head which consists of 6 to 10 **nurse cells**. The nurse cells are cortical cells which have thickened walls, enlarged nucleolus and devoid of vacuole. As the nematodes feed and reproduce, a large portion of the feeder roots are destroyed. The uptake of water and minerals are reduced and symptoms appear in the above ground tree parts.

Host range

Twenty nine species of citrus, 21 citrus hybrids and 11 species of Rutaceae are reported as hosts of this nematode. The citrus nematode has developed strains or biotype to attack grasses (*Andrapogon rhizomatus, Panicum* spp.), Olive, Grapevine, Persimmon, Pear and Lilac.

Interaction with other pathogens

The association of the nematode with *Fusarium oxysporum* and *F.solani* leads to death of plants.

Ecology

A temperature of 28-31°C has been found to be conducive for reproduction. The reproduction of nematodes is found to be good in soils of clay content of 10-15% and a pH range of 5.6 - 7.6. The slow decline symptoms are manifested in a severe form when the nematode population goes upto 40,000 juvenile / 10g of feeder roots which can be commonly seen in gardens of 12-17 years old.

Spread and survival

The mode of spread of the nematode is due to shifting of infested citrus seedling to healthy areas. Movement of soil through implements, farm labourers and animals also accounts for local spread of the nematode from one garden to the another. Spread through wind and water are also common. In soil, the nematode can remain viable in the absence of the host plant even upto 10 years.

Physiological races

Four races of *T. semipenetrans* that differ in pathogenicity to sweet orange, citrange, trifoliate orange, grapevine and lilac have been reported from different locations in California. A grass strain which infects *Andropogon rhizomatus* failed to infect citrus.

The lesion nematode *(Pratylenchus coffeae)*

Geographical distribution

P. coffeae is reported as a pest of citrus in India, Japan and USA.

Symptoms

The lesion nematodes are migratory endoparasites found in the cortical tissues of the feeder roots. Due to penetration and feeding, black lesions are produced in the cortex. These lesions gradually expand and coalesce to girdle the roots. The infected seedlings show marked reduction in root and shoot weight when compared to healthy seedlings. *Citrus limon, C.reticulata* and C. *sinensis* are commonly infested by this nematode. A temperature ranging from 10-32°C is conducive for the survival and multiplication of the nematode.

The lance nematode *(Hoplolaimus indicus)*

This nematode is an ectoparasite commonly associated with major citrus growing areas in India.

Symptoms

H. indicus reduces the plant growth of citurs. Symptoms are usually visible in 3-4 year old citrus orchards.

Life cycle

The first moult occur within the egg and the development outside the egg consists of 3 moults with 3 juvenile and the adult stage. The optimum temperature conducive for the nematode is 30°C with 16% soil moisture and pH of 7.0.

Root-knot nematode *(Meloidogyne* spp.*)*

The root-knot nematode species like *M. javanica, M. africana* and *M. indica* are recorded in citrus orchards in India. The second stage juvenile penetrates the feeder roots and fix a feeding site in root cortex. They cause characteristic root galls. The root-knot nematode causes considerable damage to citrus orchards in Andhra Pradesh when susceptible crop like tobacco or bhendi are grown as intercrops.

Management

Preventive measures

Nurseries should not be established near old orchards. The nursery soil should be sterilized before raising the seedlings. Care should be taken not to spread the nematode through tools, machineries and irrigation water.

Chemical control

a) *Bare-root dip treatment:* The seedlings can be dipped in fensulfothion, ethoprop or thionazin before planting.

b) *Soil treatment* : Granular nematicides such as carbofuran and phorate can be applied around the basin of the plant @ 1.5 kg a.i/ha. Drenching the soil around the plant with dimethoate and fensulfothion also found to be effective against the nematode.

Biological control

Incorporation of organic amendments like farmyard manure, neem cake and castor cake encourages the multiplication of predaceous nematodes (*Mononchus* spp.) which feed on the citrus nematode. Organic amendments also encourages the nematode trapping fungi of the genera *Arthrobotrys*, *Dactylella* and *Dactylaria* in citrus gardens which check the nematodes.

Resistant root stocks

Some clones and hybrids of *Poncirus trifoliata* are highly resistant to the citrus nematode. Hybridization between *Poncirus* and *Citrus* has been promising in developing resistant varieties in *Citrus* spp.

Grapevine

Grapevine is one among the important fruit crops in India. It is grown in 12,050 hectares and yielding 2,037,020 metric tonnes of fruits. It is mainly grown in Andhra Pradesh, Maharashtra, Tamil Nadu, Punjab, Haryana and Karnataka. Thompson seedless, Anab-e-Shahi, Bhokri, Bangalore Blue and Gulabi are some of the important varieties grown in India.

In India, 29 species within 15 genera of parasitic nematodes have been reported in association with grapevine. However, the root-knot nematode, *Meloidogyne incognita* and the reniform nematode, *Rotylenchulus reniformis* are the most important nematodes infesting the crop.

The root-knot nematode *(Meloidogyne incognita)*

The root-knot nematode causes yield loss upto 25 to 50 per cent. Young, shallow rooted vines are often affected by the nematodes. Nematode damage is severe when young vines are replanted in old vineyards. The cultivars such as Bangalore Blue, Gulabi and Muscat are highly susceptible to the root-knot nematode.

Geographical Distribution

The root-knot nematode is distributed in USA, Australia, Turkey and in India. In India, it has been reported from Maharashtra, Tamil Nadu, Karnataka, Andhra Pradesh, Haryana, Punjab and Delhi.

Symptoms

The affected vines show decline in vigour with inadequate sprouting even after pruning. Reduction in leaf size, marginal drying and reduction in yield are other associated symptoms. The infested roots show small galls on the roots. Heavy infestation may destroy the root systems of young plants. Root galling destroys the conducting vessels and block the flow of water and nutrients. Severe infestation leads to death of vines. The infestation is severe in light, sandy and sandyloam soils.

The Reniform nematode ***(Rotylenchulus reniformis)***

The reniform nematode is distributed in Andhra Pradesh, Uttar Pradesh, Karnataka, Maharashtra, Tamil Nadu and Delhi. It is a semi-endoparasite inserting its head and neck inside the root and exposing kidney shaped posterior body outside the root.

Management

Nematode free planting materials are to be used for raising the garden. Nematode resistant root stocks are to be used for planting.

Hot water treatment

The rootings are submerged in hot water (51.7°C) for 5 minutes. The vines are then cooled quickly and planted immediately.

Organic amendments

Neem cake can be applied @ 250 g/vine and farm yard manure can also be applied @ 2 kg/vine.

Chemical control

Soil application of carbofuran or phorate granules @ 1.5kg a.i/ha effectively checks the reniform nematode. The nematicides can be applied immediately after pruning.

Resistant root stocks

The grapevine root stocks like 1613, Dogridge and Saltcreek are resistant to the root-knot nematode. The cultivars such as Dakshi, Joazbali and Mukchilani are resistant to the reniform nematode.

Banana *(Musa* spp.*)*

Banana is the most popular fruit crop grown in the tropical and subtropical conditions. Production of the crop is affected by diseases and pests. Among the pests, the plant parasitic nematodes cause serious damage to the crop. As many as 71 species belonging to 33 genera of nematodes are in association with the crop. The most important are the burrowing nematode, *Radopholus similis*; the spiral nematode, *Helicotylenchus multicinctus*; the lesion nematode, *Pratylenchus coffeae* and the root-knot nematode, *Meloidogyne* spp.

Burrowing nematode *(Radopholus similis)*

Cobb (1893) first described the burrowing nematode from necrotic root lesions of banana in Fiji. In India the first record of the burrowing nematode was reported in Kerala during 1966. The diseases of banana caused by this nematode is known as **root rot or blackhead or blackheart or toppling disease**. The nematode causes yield loss upto 41 per cent.

Symptoms

The above ground symptoms are characterised by leaf chlorosis, dwarfing, reduction in pseudostem girth, yellowing and drying of leaves with small bunches. **'Tip over'** (sudden toppling of plants) occur even with slight wind or flood due to poor anchorage. The infected plant root and corm show characteristic reddish brown lesions due to feeding and destruction of cells (Plate 5).

Life cycle

The life cycle of burrowing nematode consists of an egg stage, four juvenile stages and an adult stage. Juveniles and females penetrate roots and feed on the cortical cells. More than one generation can occur inside the root. Males are not parasitic and have degenerated stylet.

The life cycle from egg to egg is completed in 20-25 days and females lay 4-5 eggs/day.

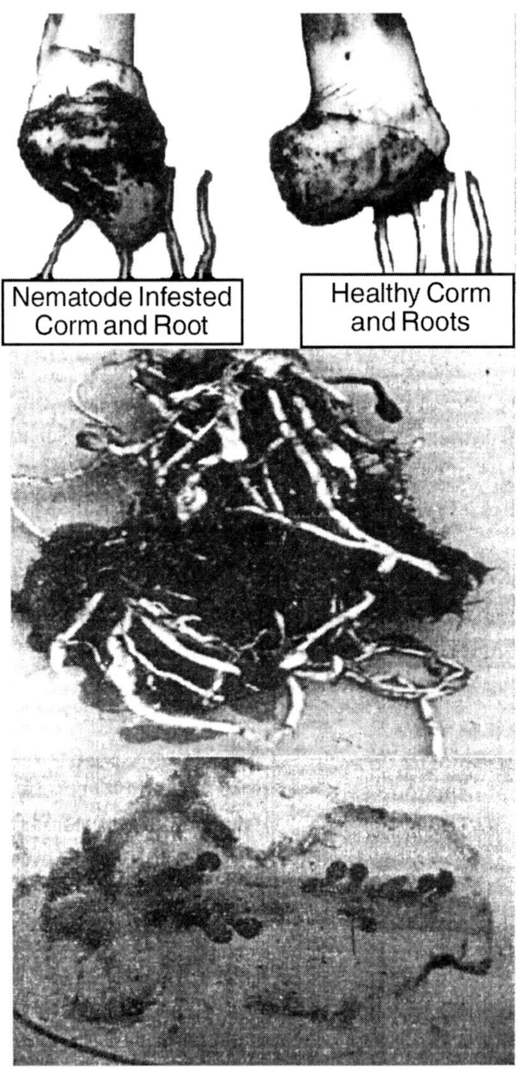

A. Banana corm and roots showing reddish brown lesion due to burrowing nematode infestation. B. Banana root showing root galls due to root-knot nematode infestation. C. Microphotograph of vertical section of a root gall showing adult females.

Plate 5: Banana infested with nematodes

Interaction with other pathogen

By wounding the host roots, the nematode provide infection site for other microorganisms. In the presence of the nematode the banana wilt menace caused by *Fusarium oxysporum* f.sp. *cubense* was doubled. Even in the wilt resistant cultivar like lacatan, breakdown of resistance was observed in the presence of the nematode.

The spiral nematode *(Helicotylenchus multicinctus)*

The spiral nematode has both endo and ectoparasitic life in banana. They are distributed in all banana growing areas. This nematode causes serious decline in bananas in the Jordan valley, Israel and India and causes yield loss upto 20 per cent.

Geographical distribution

Distributed in Israel, South Africa, Angola, Honduras, Ethiopia, Fiji, India, Malawi, Pakistan, Uganda, Brazil, Cuba, Cyprus, Ivory coast, Jamaica and Nigeria.

Symptoms

The spiral nematode causes relatively shallow necrotic lesions on banana roots and also in corms. The corm and root lesions are almost similar to that of the burrowing nematode lesions.

Life cycle

Groups of 8-26 eggs were observed in lesioned cortical tissues. Forty eight to fifty one hours are needed for the eggs to hatch in tap water at 30^{0}C. The adults and juvenile penetrate the epidermis of the root within 36 hr of inoculation. The life cycle is completed in 30-35 days.

Host range

The spiral nematode also infect cocoa, sweet potato, citrus, sugarcane, cassava, coffee, maize, mango, oil palm, rice, rubber, tea, yam, avocado and grapevine.

Lesion nematodes ***(Pratylenchus coffeae)***

Several species of lesion nematodes are known to infect banana but the most important species is *P. coffeae*. It is present in all banana growing tropical countries. The symptoms caused by *P. coffeae* are similar to the burrowing nematode. Nematodes enter the secondary roots and feed on the cortical cells, resulting in the formation of reddish brown lesions in the cortex. The nematode also infests the corms.

Life cycle

The egg to egg life cycle is completed in 27 days at 26-32°C. The optimum temperature for reproduction is 29.5°C.

Root-knot nematode *(Meloidogyne* spp.*)*

Except *M.hapla* all the other three major root-knot nematode species *viz., M. incognita, M.arenaria* and *M.javanica* readily infest banana (Jonathan *et al.,* 1999). Generally above ground symptoms are not clearly expressed. The infested plants are stuned with thin pseudostem. The galls vary in size and occur in root tips (Plate 4B).

The second stage juvenile penetrates the growing root tip and establish feeding site at vascular region. Typical multinucleate giant cells are formed 10 days after penetration. About 10-15 females are found in a single small root gall (Plate 4C). The female lays about 200-300 eggs and are deposited as egg mass in root cortex in gelatinous matrix very close to the epidermis. The life cycle is completed in 25-30 days. When the root-knot nematode is present along with Panama wilt pathogen the disease incidence will be severe in the crop.

Management

Sucker treatment

The suckers need to be selected from nematode free mother plants. The suckers can be pared to a depth of 1cm and treated in hot water (55°C for 10 minutes) or in monocrotophos 36 EC 0.5% solution for 10 minutes prior to planting.

Paring and pralinage treatment

The suckers selected from mother plants are pared to a depth of 1 cm, dipped in mud slurry and 40g of carbofuran 3G is spread all over the corm and planted in soil.

Crop rotation

In wetland the banana crop can be rotated with rice crop.

Intercrops

Marigold (*Tagetes* spp.) can be grown in between suckers and incorporated around the plants. The alfa terthenyl compounds present in marigold plant kills the nematodes.

Organic amendments

Neem cake, farm yard manure and pressmud can be applied to encourage the predacious nematodes and antagonistic fungi which in turn kill the nematodes.

Resistant varieties

Bodles Altaport is found to be resistant to *R.similis*.

Papaya

Papaya (*Carica papaya*) is an important tropical and sub-tropical fruit crop grown in an area of 34,000 hectares in India. Papain, a proteolytic enzyme extracted from the fruit is used in pharmaceutical, cosmetics, textile, paint and meat-industries.

The root-knot (*Meloidogyne incognita*) and reniform (*Rotylen-chulus reniformis*) nematodes cause serious damage to the crop. Growth and vigour are reduced and severe infestation leads to premature death of trees. Studies indicated 20-40 per cent yield loss in the crop due to nematode infestation.

Root-knot nematode *(Meloidogyne incognita)*

The second stage juveniles of the root-knot nematode penetrates the growing root tip and fixes a feeding site in the cortex as a sedentary endoparasite. The nematode matures in 20-25 days and lays about 200-300 eggs in a gelatinous matrix on the infested root. Due to continuous feeding, histopathological changes occur in the cortical parenchyma cells, resulting in the formation of giant cells. Proliferation of cells also takes place in the cortex due to hypertrophy and hyperplasia by repeated mitosis. These histopathological changes create a pressure inside the root cells, causing dislocation of xylem vessels leading to impaired translocation of water and minerals to the aerial parts.

Symptoms

The characteristic symptoms are stunted growth, yellowing of leaves and day wilt even with adequate moisture in soil. Infested plant roots are malformed due to severe root galling (Plate 6).

Reniform nematode *(R. reniformis)*

The reniform nematode usually penetrate the secondary and tertiary roots and causes necrotic lesions. The female is attached to the root as a semiendoparasite with its posterior kidney shaped body protruding outside the root (Plate 7). An adult female lays 50-75 eggs in gelatinous matrix. Apart from this direct damage, injuries caused to the roots due to penetration by the nematodes facilitate easy entry of soil borne fungal pathogens *viz., Phytophthora* and *Fusarium*, causing root rot disease.

Management

Summer ploughing and exposing the soil to sun light for one or two months during April-May prior to planting help to reduce the nematode and pathogen load in the soil.

Selection of nematode free papaya seedlings for planting (Discard seedlings having galled and decayed root system.)

Application of farmyard manure, neem cake, pressmud and carbofuran 3G at 8kg, 100g, 3kg and 33g respectively per plant at the time of planting in the pit.

Prophylactic drenching with Bordeaux mixture at 0.1 per cent at monthly intervals during the north-east monsoon period.

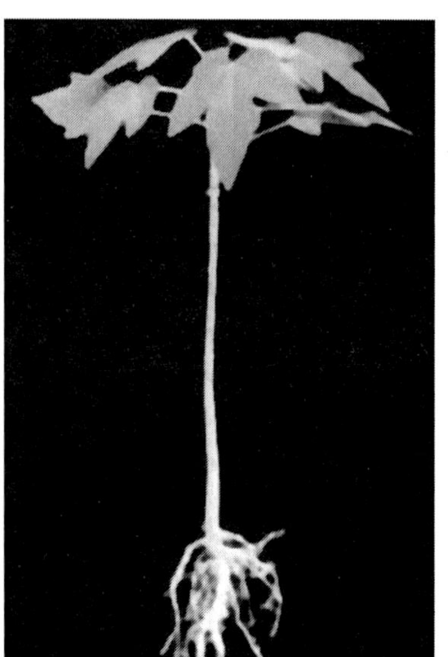

Plate 6: Papaya seedling infested with root-knot nematode

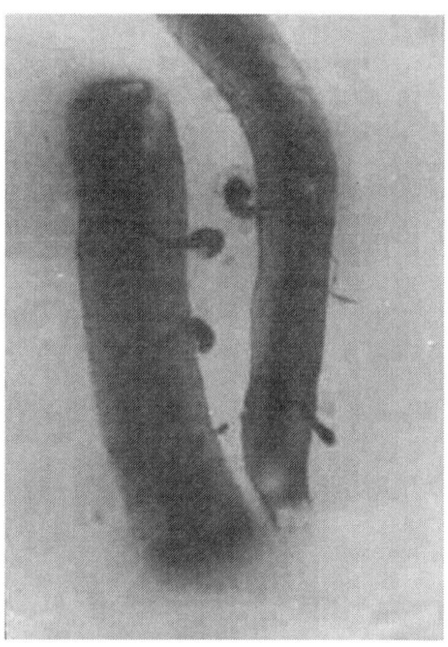

Plate 7: Papaya root infested with reniform nematode (reniform females attached to the root as semiendoparasite)

Provision of good drainage and avoidance of water stagnation.

Rotating papaya crop with marigold helps to reduce the nematode incidence for the next crop.

12

Nematode Pests of Vegetable Crops

Potato

Potato is one of the most important vegetable crop grown in India. It thrives best in cool climate. Therefore it is a summer crop in the hills and a winter crop in plains.

Twenty seven species of nematodes have been reported on potato among them the cyst nematodes (*Globodera rostochiensis* and *G. pallida*) and the root-knot nematodes (*Meloidogyne incognita, M. javanica* and *M. hapla*) are important in India.

Cyst nematodes *(G.rostochiensis and G. pallida)*

In India, the cyst nematode menace on potato was first reported by Dr. Jones during 1961 from Nilgiri Hills.

Geographical distribution

The potato cyst nematode is distributed in Central, South and North America, Europe, Iceland, Western USSR and South Africa.

In India it is distributed in Nilgiri and Kodai Hills and in New Delhi.

Symptoms

The severely infested plants are stunted and show day wilting during hot part of the day. The symptoms occur in patches. Plants show tufting of leaves on the top and the outer leaves show yellowing and subsequently die. Root system is smothered and secondary roots are induced. Such plants can be easily pulled out. Such plants can be easily pulled out. Tubers formed are small and less in number. In severe infestation tuber formation is arrested.

Life cycle

G.rostochiensis is amphimictic with sessile and globose females. The males are vermiform. The second stage juvenile is the resistant, dormant and infective stage remaining inside the egg within the cyst formed by tanning of female cuticle. The cysts remain in the soil after death of the host. Each cyst usually contain about 300-500 eggs. After hatching, the second stage juveniles enter the host root just behind the root tip or at the site of new lateral root and move to the cortex of pericycle region and fix feeding site. The feeding site consist of 4 to 6 syncytial transfer cells on which the nematode feeds and develop into an adult. The adult female swells, rupturing the cortex and protrudes from the root, exposing the vulval region outside while the head and neck remain inserted in the root (Plate 8). The adult females are initially white in colour known as **white female** and later on, due to quinone tanning, the cuticle becomes leathery cyst which are dark brown in colour. In case of root-knot of nematode infestation root galls are produced in the root (Plate 9).

Host range

All known varieties of potato, tomato and brinjal are attacked by the cyst nematode. A number of species which come under the genus *Solanum* are hosts of the nematode. The only susceptible plant outside the family is Snapdragon and *Antirrhinum majus*.

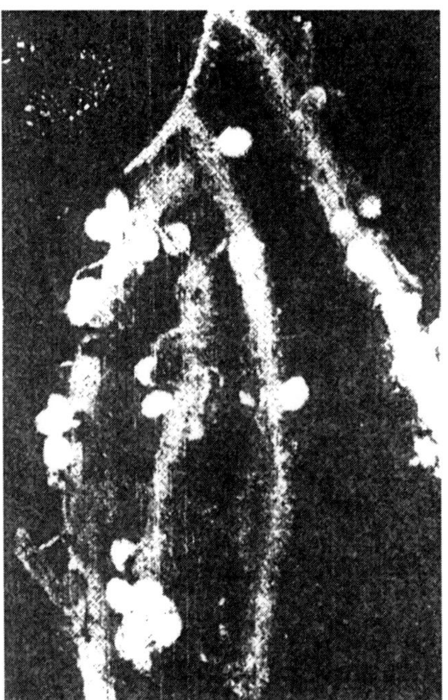

Plate 8: Potato root showing white females protruding the root

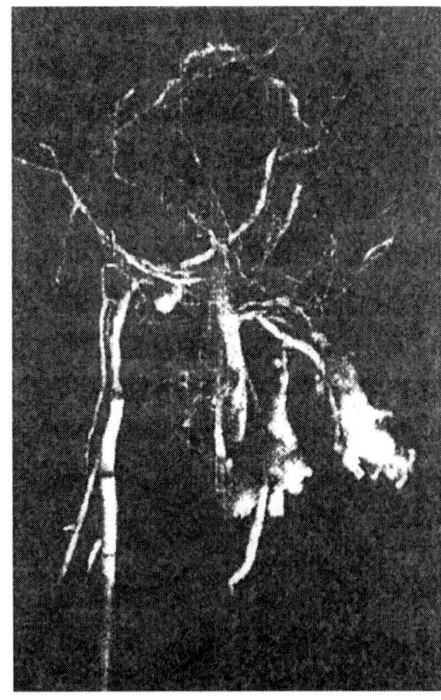

Plate 9: Potato root showing root galls due to root-knot nematode infestation

Interaction with other pathogen

The potato cyst nematode and the fungus, *Rhizoctonia solani* cause great loss when both the organisms are found together. The nematode also interact with *Verticillium dahliae* and enhance the severity of the wilt disease. *G.pallida* is reported to have an association with *Pseudomonas solanacearum*.

Spread and survival

The cysts can remain viable in the soil without the host even upto 30 years. The cysts can spread through the displacement of soil along with seed material for a very long distance. Movement of farm machineries and tools helps to carry the infested soil along with them. The cyst being very light in weight can be easily carried by wind to a long distance.

Management

Cultural control

Growing non-host crops like wheat, maize, beans etc. Following crop rotation for one year with non-solanaceous vegetables such as peas, cabbage, cauliflower and carrot during autumn season reduces the cyst nematode.

Quarantine

The infested area should be quarantined and seed material should not be allowed to move out of the infested areas. Volunteer seedlings in the infested area should be destroyed.

Resistant varieties

Solanum vernei and *S. tuberosum* sp. *andigena* were found to have resistance against the cyst nematode of potato. Roots of these plants are readily invaded by infective juveniles, which however fail to mature and reproduce because the root tissues are not induced to produce giant cells and thus the female cannot develop. **Kufri Swarna** is a cyst nematode resistant hybrid potato released by Central Potato Research Institute during the year 1986.

Chemical control

Aldicarb @ 2kg. a.i/ha as spot treatment was found to be the economical and effective method of control.

Nematode pests on other vegetable crops

A large number of plant parasitic nematodes have been recorded from the rhizosphere of many other vegetable crops. An yield loss of 91, 46 and 27 per cent have been recorded in bhendi, tomato and brinjal respectively, due to the root-knot nematode, *Meloidogyne spp.*

Root-knot nematode (*Meloidogyne* spp.)

The first record of root-knot nematode was made by Berkeley during 1855 in cucumber. Almost all the vegetable crops have been found to be susceptible to the root-knot nematode species, *M.incognita* and *M.javanica* are found in warmer areas of the plains where as *M.hapla* is specific to the temperate region.

The vegetable crops like bhendi, brinjal, tomato, carrot, radish, chillies, cauliflower, cabbage, gourds and garden beans are often infected by this nematode (Plate 10 &11).

The second stage juveniles penetrate the young roots behind the root cap and migrate to cortex region and fix a feeding site. At the feeding site 4-5 giant cells are formed which provide nourishment to the developing juveniles. The giant cells are bigger in size and multinucleate with dense cytoplasm. At the feeding site proliferation of cells occur due to hypertrophy and hyperplasia. Due to pressure in the cortical tissue, galls are formed on the roots. The gall formation leads to the destruction of xylem vessels which in turn affects conduction of water and the nutrients to the above ground parts. The adult female lays 200-300 eggs in a gelatinous matrix which usually protrudes outside the roots. The life cycle is normally completed in 25-30 days depending upon the host and other ecological factors. The infested plants show yellowing and stunting of plants. In severe infestation premature death of plants are also noticed. The size and intensity of root galls caused by the root-knot nematode vary according to the nematode species and the host plant. In tomato and bhendi, *M.incognita* produces very big root galls on severe infestation (Plate 12 &13).

Apart from their direct damage, the minute injuries caused by the nematode have way for other soil borne pathogens like *Fusarium*, *Phytophthora*, *Rhizoctonia* and *Verticillium* enhance the disease caused by the organisms.

Reniform nematode (*Rotylenchulus reniformis*)

Reniform nematode is a semi-endoparasite and causes damage to beans, cabbage, carrot, cauliflower, cucumber, brinjal, pea, cowpea, radish, bhendi and lettuce. The preadult females are parasitic. The nematode initiate infection by destroying the epidermal cells and cause necrosis. Disintegration of phloem cells occur in the stelar region of plants. Juveniles of female survive for six months in desiccated soil and for several months in moist soil. The fourth stage juveniles are better adapted to adverse condition. The adult females are reniform in shape with their head and neck inside the root whereas the posterior reniform shaped body seen outside the root. The female lays 150-200 eggs in gelations matrix.

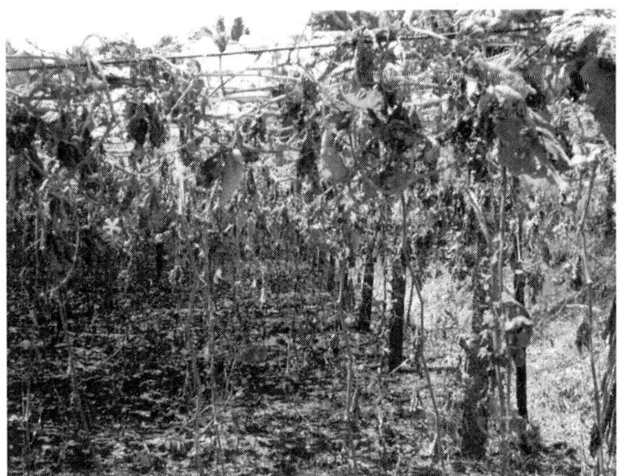

Plate 10: Root knot nematode infested snakegourd field

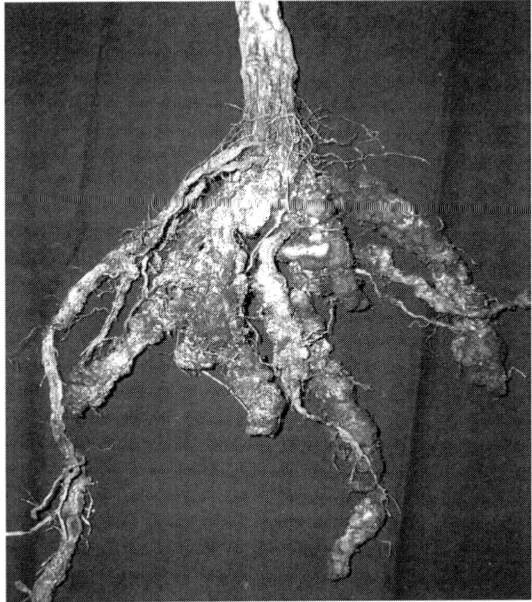

Plate 11: Snakegourd roots showing severe galls

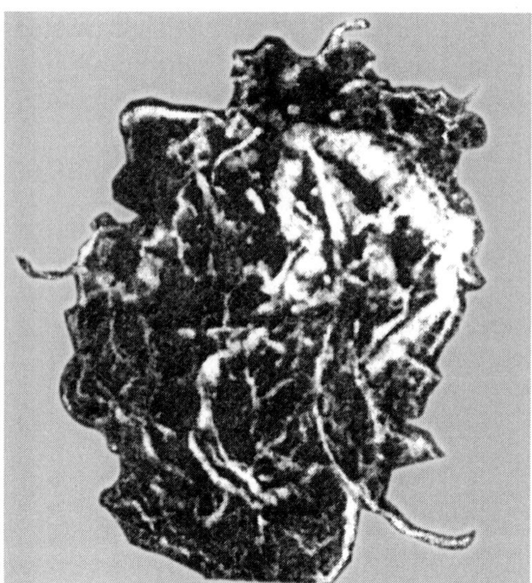

Plate 12: Tomato root showing severe root galls due to root-knot nematode infestation

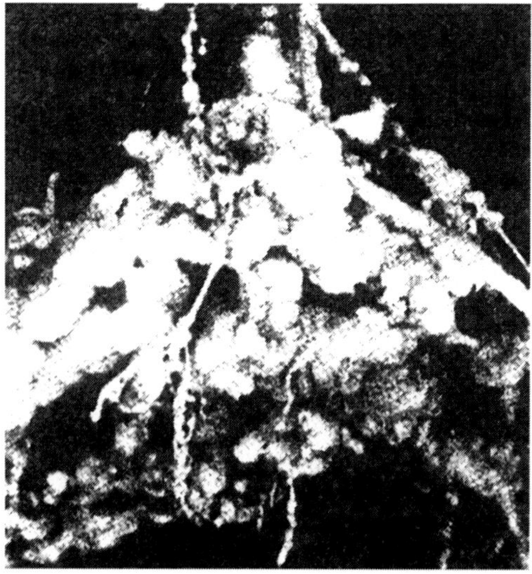

Plate 13: Bhendi root showing severe root galls due to root-knot nematode infestation

Stem and bulb nematode (*Ditylenchus* spp.)

The stem nematode commonly attack beans, peas, carrot, potato onion and garlic.

D.dipsaci commonly feeds on stems, leaves and bulbs and very rarely found in soil. It penetrates the germinating seed and lives in the parenchyma tissues beneath the hilum in cotyledons. The infected seedling become stunted, twisted, enlarged and malformed. The foliage collapse and softening of the bulb begins at the neck and gradually proceeds downward. The life cycle is completed in 19-23 days. The nematode has got an adaptation to form **"nematode wool"** to escape from desiccation stress.

Stunt nematode (*Tylenchorhynchus* spp.)

The most common species of stunt nematode is *T. brassicae* which cause damage to cabbage and cauliflower in Uttar Pradesh. The seedling growth is very much reduced due to the nematode. The nematode is mostly an ectoparasite and rarely observed in the stelar region. The multiplication of the nematode takes place in a wide range of temperature (15-35°C).

Management

The nursery needs to be raised in nematode free soil. Nematode infested seedlings should not be used for planting. Soil solarisation in nursery beds using polythene sheets during summer reduces the soil infestation of nematodes. Soil solarisation is an effective measure for vegetable crops raised in the nursery beds.

Rotation of crops like tomato, brinjal, bhendi and chilli with non hosts crops like mustard, sesame, maize, wheat and rice.

Use of organic amendments

Incorporation of decomposed farm yard manure, poultry manure and green leaf manures reduce the nematode infestation by promoting the predaceous nematodes and other antagonistic fungi which checks the parasitic nematodes. During decomposition of organic matter, several organic acids, ammonia and other nematode toxic compounds are released in soil.

Chemical Treatment

Nursery beds can be treated with carbofuran 3G @ 0.3g a.i/m^2. In mainfield, carbofuran or phorate can be applied as spot treatment @ 1.5 kg a.i./ha on 15 days after transplanting.

Host plant resistance

The use of resistant varieties proved an effective, economical and friendly means of nematode control. Hissar Lalit and NDTR are resistant tomatoes against *Meloidogyne spp.* Pusa Jwala is a resistant chilli variety against *M. incognita.*

13

Nematode Pests of Commercial Flower Crops

Crossandra

Crossandra (*Crossandra undulaefolia*) is one of the important commercially grown flower crop in Tamil Nadu. In recent years there is a marked decline in the cultivation of this crop in Madurai, Dindigul, Coimbatore, Salem, Thiruvannamalai and Tiruchirappalli districts. The common problem with the crop is death of plants in patches during the second and third year. This is due to the nematode-fungal complex disease in the crop.

Investigations revealed the association of root-knot nematode, *Meloidogyne* spp. and the root-lesion nematode, *Pratylenchus delattrei* with the crop along with fungal patheogen, *Fusarium solani.*

Root-knot nematode

Both *M. incognita* and *M. javanica* are reported to cause damage and yield loss to the crop. The affected plants exhibit stunted growth, yellowing of leaves and also have chlorotic symptoms. The nematode in association with *R. solani* causes serious damage to the crop. The infested plants show root galls.

Root-lesion nematode

The root-lesion nematode, *P. delattrei* causes serious damage to the crop and prevalent in all the localities where the crop is continuously cultivated. This is a migratory endoparasite and causes damage to the cortical parenchyma cells in the root. The infested root shows brown to black colour lesions varying in length and intensity.

The affected plant leaves exhibit mottled appearance and pink colouration which ultimately turn yellow and wither.

Nematode fungal complex disease

The association of the nematode and wilt disease pathogen *Rhizoctonia* and *Fusarium* leads to mortially of plants. The disease incidence will be more if both the nematode and the pathogen are found together in the field.

Management of the nematode fungal complex disease

Planting nematode free healthy seedlings in the main field. Treating the nursery bed with phorate 10G @ 5g / m^2 Application of neem cake @ 100g / m^2

The nursery beds needs to be drenched with 0.1% carbendazim solution one week after nematicide application.

In the main field spot application of phorate 10G @ 1g / plant on 30 days after transplanting and one week after nematicide application; spot drenching with carbendazim at 0.1% is done to manage the nematode fungal complex disease in the crop.

Tuberose

Tuberose (*Polyanthes tuberosa*) is a valued commercial flower crop for its prettiness, elegance and sweet pleasant fragrance. It has got a great economic potential for cut flower trade and essential oil industry. It is cultivated in the tropical and subtropical countries of the world. The flowers are used for artistic garlands, floral ornaments, bouquets and buttonholes (Plate 14A). The flowers emit a delightful fragrance and are the source of tuberose oil. In India, it is cultivated in West Bengal, Karnataka, Tamil Nadu and Maharastra.

Many plant parasitic nematodes are reported from the rhizosphere of tuberose. Among them the root-knot nematode, *Meloidogyne incognita* and *M. javanica* are commonly associated with the crop and cause serious damage. The infested plants show yellowing and drying up of leaves. Stunting of plants also occur in patches (Plate 14B). In case of severe infestation the spike emergence is suppressed resulting in loss of flower yield. Emergence of side shoots from bulbs were also seen in some plants. The infested plant root have characteristic root galls of varying size (Plate 14C).

Management

Summer ploughing and exposing the field to sunlight during the month of May for a period of one month prior to planting the bulbs, minimize the initial nematode load in the soil. Spot application of phorate 10G or carbofuran 3 G @ 1 kg a.i / ha. is also effective. Addition of farm yard manure @ 30 t / ha enhance the multiplication of predacious nematodes and antagonistic fungi which inturn checks the plant parasitic nematode in the crop.

Jasmine

Jasmine (*Jasminum sambac*) is an important commercial flower crop grown mainly in countries like India, China and Malaysia. The natural oil of jasmine is used in high grade perfumes. The crop is grown in an area of 1025 ha in Tamil Nadu.

Many plant parasitic nematodes are reported from the rhizosphere of the crop. Among them few are very important. The root-knot nematode, *Meloidogyne incognita*; the lesion nematode *Pratylenchus delattrei* and the spiral nematode, *Helicotylenchus* spp. are often associated with the crop.

The root-knot nematode infested jasmine plant root show characteristic galls. The second stage juveniles of the nematode penetrate the growing root tip and invade the cortical parenchyma cells. The nematode fix feeding site in root cortex and develop to become adult. The adult female lays 200-300 eggs. The life cycle is completed in 25-30 days.

The lesion nematodes are migratory endoparasites invading the roots and destroy the cortical cells. This leads to dark lesions on the root surface and subsequently rotting of roots occur and then the nematode migrate to invade fresh healthy roots. The infested plants show stunted growth and yellowing of leaves. The jasmine plants of more than two years age are commonly infested by these nematodes.

Nematode fungal complex disease

Soil borne fungal pathogen (*Fusarium* spp.) easily enter the root through the injuries caused by the nematodes. Thus the nematode act as a pre-disposing factor for the severe wilt disease in jasmine crop.

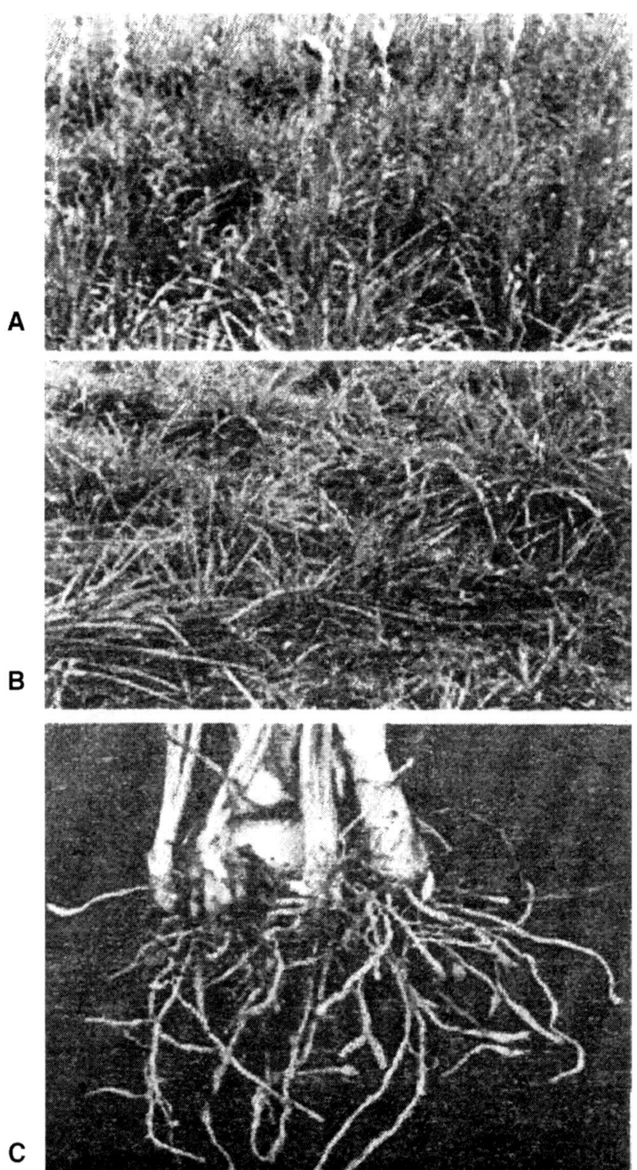

Plate 14: A. Healthy Tuberose plot B. Root-knot nematode infested Tuberose plot C. Tuberose root showing severe root galls due to M. incognita infestation

Management of nematode fungal complex disease

Summer ploughing and exposing the field to sunlight during the month of May for a period of one month prior to planting, minimize the initial nematode and soil borne fungal pathogen in soil. Spot application of phorate 10g 5g/plant or carbofuran 3G @ 15g/plant. Addition of farm yard manure @ 5 kg/plant to enhance the multiplication of predacious nematodes and nematophagous fungi which inturn checks the plant parasitic nematodes in the crop. Spot drenching is also done with carbendazim at 0.1 per cent, one week after nematicide application. The granular nematicide and carbendazim treatment have to be given once in every six months in order to arrest the nematode and pathogen multiplication.

14

Nematode Pests of Spice and Plantation Crops

Black Pepper

Black pepper (*Piper nigrum*) is indigenous to the tropical forests of Western Ghats of South India. The crop is grown in Kerala, Karnataka, Tamil Nadu, Andra Pradesh and Assam.

The root-knot nematode, *Meloidogyne incognita* and the burrowing nematode, *Radopholus similis* are important pests of this crop. The root-knot nematode infested vines show yellowing of lower leaves and the leaves loose natural luster. The yellowing of leaves gradually progresses upwards. The affected vine leaves become flaccid and wither. The infested plant root show root galls of varying sizes.

The burrowing nematode also causes serious damage to the vine. Var der Vecht (1950) first reported slow wilt in this crop due to *R.similis* infestation in Indonesia. The nematode in association with *Fusarium* and *Rhizoctonia* causes serious damage to the crop.

Management

Treat the plants in the nursery with carbofuran 3G @ 1.5 kg a.i/ha. In the main field the vines can be treated once in 6 months with carbofuran @ 1.5-2.0 kg a.i/ha. Application of neem cake @ 0.5 to 1 kg / vine also reduce the nematode damage.

Cardamom

Cardamom (*Elettaria cardamomum*) is native of evergreen rainy forests of Western Ghats in South India. It is cultivated in Kerala, Karnataka and Tamil Nadu. Cardamom is used for flavouring various preparations of food, confectionery and beverages.

The root-knot nematode, *Meloidogyne* spp; reniform nematode, *R. reniformis*; root lesion nematode, *Pratylenchus* spp. and the burrowing nematode, *R.similis* have been reported pathogenic to this crop.

The nematode damage causes yellowing and stunting of plants in nursery and manifield. In case of severe infestation shedding of immature capsules are observed. The plants infested with root-knot nematode have root galls and abnormal branching of roots.

Management

The nurseries can be treated with carbofuran 3G @ 1.5 kg a.i/ha and in the manifield the nematiciede needs to be applied once in 6 months.

Turmeric

Turmeric (*Curcuma longa*) is grown in the states of Andhra Pradesh, Maharastra, Tamil Nadu, Orissa, Kerala and Bihar. It is a herbaceous perennial with a thick underground rhizome giving rise to primary and secondary rhizomes called fingers.

The root-knot nematode, *Meloidogyne* spp. is widely prevalent in all the turmeric grown areas. The nematodes are spread through the rhizomes. In case of severe infestation stunting and yellowing of plants appear in patches. The infested plant root show severe root galls and there will be poor development of fingers.

Management

Application of carbofuran 3G or phorate 10G @ 1-1.5 kg a.i/ha. Neem cake application @ 1 t/ha also reduces the nematode incidence.

Arecanut

Arecanut (*Areca catechu*) is primarily grown for its kernel obtained from the fruit. It is grown in countries like India, Bangladesh and Sri Lanka. In India the crop is grown in Kerala, Karnataka, Assam and Tamil Nadu. In recent years there is a decline in production due to number of pests and diseases. Association of plant parasitic nematodes is also one of the reasons for decline in yield. About 22 genera of parasitic nematodes are reported to be associated with the rhizosphere of the crop. The burrowing nematode, *Radopholus similis* is the only important nematode which cause significant damage to the crop.

Symptoms of damage

R. similis is a migratory endoparasite and causes lesions and rotting on root. The nematode produce elongate orange coloured lesions on the young and succulent root. The lesions coalesce and cause rotting of root. The thick primary roots from the bole region of the plant may have oval sunken brown lesions. The nematode invade the cortex by inter and interacellularly. In the nematode infested plant the root system is very much reduced (Plate 15). The nematode lays eggs in the cavities in root cortex. The nematode complete its life cycle in 25-30 days. The nematode in association with the fungus, *Cylindrocarpon obtusisporum* causes extensive damage to the crop.

Management

Treating the grown up trees with phorate 10G or carbofuran 3G @ 10g a.i/ palm was found to reduce the nematode infestation.

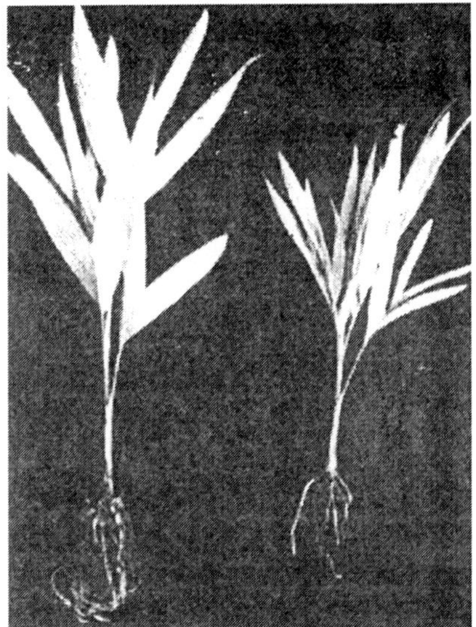

Healthy seedling Nematode infested

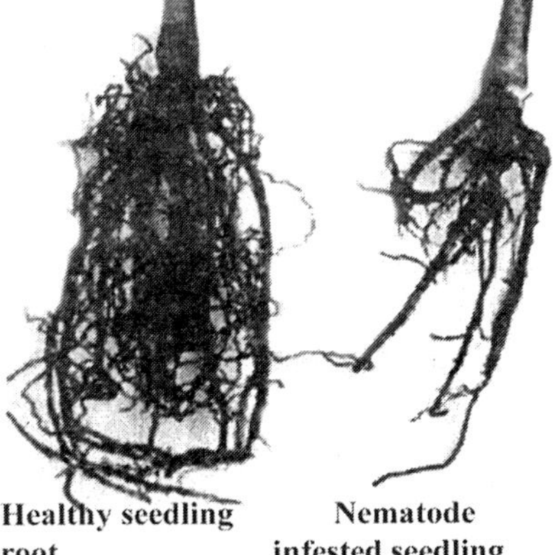

Plate 15: Arecanut (Healthy and *R. similis* infested) seedlings

Coffee

The lesion nematode, *Pratylenchus coffeae* is an important pest of coffee in India. *P. coffeae* destroyed 95 per cent of arabica coffee plantations in Java. The annual loss due to this nematode was estimated at 3 million dollars.

Geographical distribution

Distributed in Dominican Republic, E1 Salvador, Guatemala, India, Indonesia and Venezuela. Over 10,000 hectares have been infested with this nematode in coffee growing tracts of South India.

Symptoms

In nurseries, the lesion nematode causes death of plants. The infested plants show yellowing of leaves, stunting and gradual wilting which follows death of plants. The infested plants can be easily pulled out by hand because of poor root growth. On closer observation, lesion can be seen on the root.

Life cycle

P. coffeae is a migratory endoparasite of the root cortex where it feeds and multiplies. The nematode invades the growing root tip at the elongation zone. A colony of nest can be seen in the lesioned root tissue. When the lesioned root decay, the nematodes migrate to invade fresh root. The first moult takes place within the egg and three moults occur outside. The life cycle is completed in 45 to 48 days. The eggs hatch out in 15 to 17 days, remain 15 to 16 days as juveniles and takes 15 days from maturity to egg production.

Host range

P. coffeae is known to attack coffee, banana, citrus, grapevine, apples, strawberry, abaca, yam, cocoa, rubber, potato, sweet potato, peas, beans, cabbage, cauliflower, tomato, chrysanthemum, caladium, dahlia, marigold, cotton and lucerne.

Management

Resistant rootstocks

Coffea robusta is resistant to *P. coffeae* than *C. arabica.* Coffee varieties susceptible to *P. coffeae* can be successfully grafted on nematode-resistant root stocks such as *C. conuga* and *C. robusta.*

Organic amendments

Coffee pulp at 18 kg/m^2 improves plant growth and reduces the nematode infestation.

Nematicides

Aldicarb or carbofuran or phorate can be applied @ 1.5 kg a.i/ha as ring application around the coffee plants.

Tea

Root-knot nematodes, *Meloidogyne* spp. are the most important nematodes in tea plantations and causes damage to the crop. Twenty one species of nematodes belonging to 14 genera have been reported in association with tea crop in India.

Nematode damage in young tea

Barber (1901) first reported severe infestation of *M. javanica, M. incognita* and *M. hapla* in South India. Young nursery plants, both seedlings and vegetatively propagated clonal plants are severely damaged by root-knot nematodes. In seedlings both tap root and lateral roots are severely infested than the clonal tea plants and it is due to very less root growth in seedlings plants. A marked increase in resistance is observed between 8 and 15 months.

Nematodes on mature tea

M. brevicauda causes severe galling of the roots of mature tea bushes and causes decline in growth and vigour of the plant. Tea plants of all ages are susceptible to infection by this nematode. This problem is found in Sri Lanka and India.

The infected bushes grow slowly and produce small leaves which turn yellow. The roots show characteristic swelling and pitting which is typical of *M. brevicauda* damage. The effect of infection on the growth of tea bushes is evident during the period of recovery from pruning. Healthy bushes are usually harvested in about 16 weeks after pruning and it is delayed by 6 months in infested plants. The most severely affected bushes fail to recover from pruning.

Management

Raise nurseries in nematode free soil. Fumigants such as EDB can be used to disinfect the nursery soil.

Fesulfothion 5G at 14g/plant gives effective control of the root-knot nematodes.

Incorporation of organic matter in the form of farm yard manure and neem cake reduce the incidence of the nematodes.

Pre-plant cultivation of marigold reduces the infestation of root- knot nematodes

Betelvine

Betelvine is cultivated in Orissa, Andhra Pradesh, Tamil Nadu, Kerala, Karnataka, Maharastra, Madhya Pradesh, Assam, Uttar Pradesh and Bihar. About 40 species of plant parasitic nematodes are associated with the crop in India. Among them, the most important and frequently observed nematodes are *Meloidogyne incognita*, *Rotylenchulus reniformis* and *Helocotylenchus incisus.* The root-knot nematode causes typical root galls in the betelvine root (Plate 16).

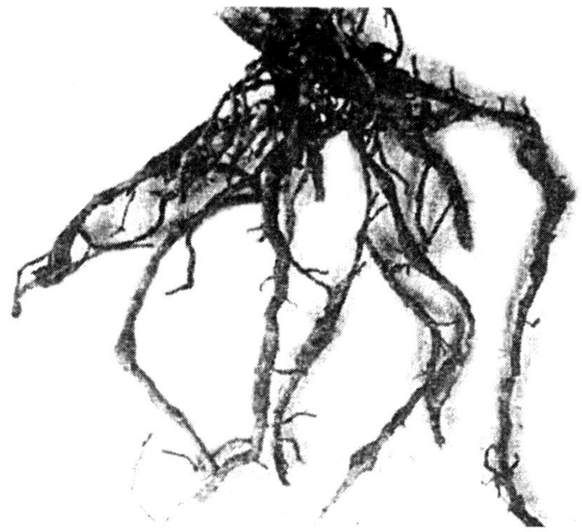

Plate 16: Betelvine root showing severe root galls due to root-knot nematode infestation

The reniform nematode, *R. reniformis* is a semi-endoparasite and causes lesions on the root. This nematode also enhance the wilt disease in association with *Phytophthora* spp. The adult female can be seen in the infested root. The reniform shaped females protrude their posterior body outside where as the head and neck are embedded inside the cortical tissue (Plate 17).

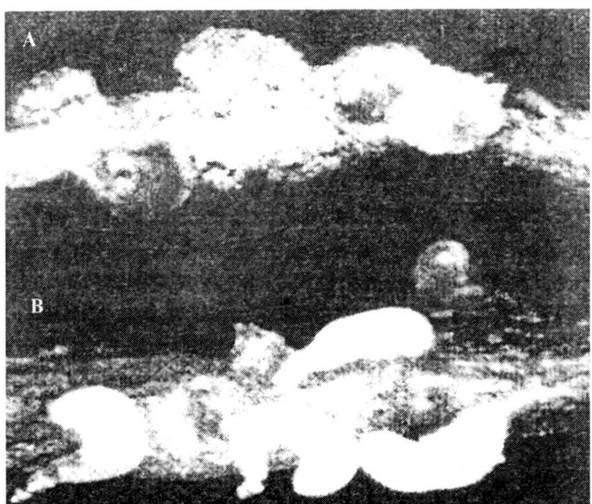

Plate 17: A. Reinform nematode females attached to the betelvine root covered with egg masses. **B.** Reinform shaped females attached to the betelvine root

The spiral nematode, *Helicotylenchus incisus* is an ectoparasite and feed on the growing root tip. They cause lesions on the root.

Management

Application of farm yard manure @ 30 t/ha. Application of neem cake @ 3 t/ha in three split doses at 45 days interval along with manures.

Spot application of the parasitic fungus, *Paecilomyces lilacinus* inoculated neem cake @ 500 kg/ha at the rhizosphere of the vine at quarterly interval was found to be very effective in controlling the root knot and reniform nematodes.

Since, the leaves are used for chewing, nematicides are not recommended for the betelvine crop, considering the residual toxicity problem.

Nematode pests of medicinal and aromatic plants

In the recent years there has been an increased interest in the cultivation of medicinal and aromatic plants to meet the requirement of cosmetics, flavouring, perfumery and pharmaceutical industries and also to earn foreign exchange by way of export. Plant parasitic nematodes associated with these crops affect their yield quantitatively and qualitatively. Hence proper attention has to be given for the management of nematodes affecting these medicinal and aromatic plants.

Nematode of Dioscorea spp.

Yams, *Dioscorea* spp are probably one of the oldest food crops known to man besides their medicinal value. Several nematode species have been found associated with *Dioscorea* spp. The nematodes of particular importance are endoparasites of roots and tubers. Those known to cause serious damage are *Scutellonema bradys*, *Pratylenchus coffeae* and *Meloidogyne* spp.

Scutellonema bradys

The yam nematode *S. bradys* causes the decay of yam tubers known as 'dry rot disease'.

Symptoms

- Cream and light yellow lesions below the outer skin of the tuber as initial symptoms and there are no external symptoms at this stage.
- As the disease progresses it spreads into the tuber normally to a maximum depth of 2 cm but sometimes deeper.
- In the later stages of dry rot, infected tissues are first observed as light brown and subsequently become dark brown to black; external cracks appear in the skin of the tubers and parts can flake off exposing patches of dark brown, dry rot tissues.

Pratylenchus coffeae

Symptoms

- Infected plants are shorter and unthrifty besides showing general symptoms of nematode damage.
- Brown, irregular dry rot extending upto 1 – 2 cm into the outer tissues of tubers.

Meloidogyne spp.

Symptoms

- Galling of yam roots. Foliar symptoms includes early yellowing, leaf withering and termination of plant growth.

Management

- Fallowing
- Grow non - host (or) poor hosts such as maize or sorghum prior to yams

- Crops which are known to support high nematode population should be avoided. Eg. Cowpea
- Use of nematode free seed material
- Hot water treatment of tubers (50 – 55°C for 40 min)
- Use of carbofuran @ 1 kg a.i/ha.

Nematodes of Patchouli

Patchouli (*Pogostemon cablin* Benth. Syn. P. *patchouli* Pallet. Var. sauvis Hook) is native of the Phillipines and grows in India, Indonesia, Malaysia and Singapore. The essential oil of patchouli is used commercially in the perfumery industries of the world as a base because of its fixative property. The patchouli oil is also used in Ayurvedic medicine to treat nausea, diarrhoea, cold and headache. The patchouli oil is extensively used in food industries as flavour ingredient. The most important nematodes which severely affect the crop are *Meloidogyne incognita, M. javanica, M. hapla* and *Pratylenchus brachyurus.*

Symptoms of Damage

Heavy galling on the root system due to infestation of root knot nematode on patchouli results in stunting, wilting, defoliation and yellowing of the plant. Sometimes root galls are very small (2 mm) or the surrounding galls coalesce to form a larger one. The infection of root knot nematode occurs when the plants are in their early stage of growth.

Management of Nematodes of Patchouli

- Control of *Meloidogyne incognita* on patchouli was obtained by application of Carbofuran @ 1kg a.i. / ha as pre or post plant treatment.
- Application of different oil seed cakes such as neem, pongamia and castor improved the plant growth and reduced the nematode population.
- Application of neem oil seed cakes @ 4 tonnes / ha proved better than other oilseed cakes for increasing the growth and yield of the crop and reducing the *M.incognita* population.
- Summer fallowing also proved a good method for reducing *M. incognita* population below threshold levels.
- Application of aldicarb, carbofuran or phorate @ 2 or 3 kg a.i. / ha to control *Helicotylenchus dihystera* on *patchouli.*

Nematodes of Geranium

Geranium (*Pelargonium graveolens* L.) is one of the important source of an expensive essential oil used in high grade soap, perfumery and cosmotic industries because of rosy aroma. The important constituents of its oil are 1 - isomenthone, isoamyl alcohol and methyl pentanol. It is also a source of rhodinol. The root knot nematode, M. *incognita, M. hapla* and the spiral nematode, *Helicotylenchus* sp. cause serious damage to the crop.

Symptoms of Damage

Root knot nematode infested plants generally show stunting, burning of lower leaves, yellowing and severe galling on the root system. *M.incognita* and *M. hapla* are the most important nematode pathogens associated with the decline of crop yield. Reduction upto 50% of oil yield of geranium due to *M. incognita, M. hapla* has been reported.

Management of Nematodes in Geranium

- Application of aldicarb, carbofuran, phorate and quinalphos @ 2 or 3 kg a.i./ ha after four months of transplanting the cuttings of the plants.
- Aldicarb @ 3 kg a.i. / ha effectively controlled the population of *Scutellonema conicephalum, Meloidogyne hapla* and *Helicotylenchus dihystera* and increased the foliage and oil yield of geranium.

15

Nematode Control

Nematode Control

Plant parasitic nematodes can be controlled by several methods. The nematode control aims to improve growth, quality and yield by keeping the nematode population below the economical threshold level. The control measures to be adopted should be profitable and cost effective. It is essential to calculate the cost benefit ratio before adopting control measures.

The nematode control methods are

1. Regulatory (Legal) control
2. Physical control
3. Cultural control
4. Biological control
5. Chemical control

1. Regulatory Control

Regulatory control of pests and diseases is the legal enforcement of measures to prevent them from spreading or having spread, from multiplying sufficiently to become intolerably troublesome. The principle involved in enacting quarantine is exclusion of nematode from entering into an area which is not infested in order to avoid spread of the nematode.

Quarantine principles are traditionally employed to restrict the movement of infected plant materials and contaminated soil into a state or country. Many countries maintain elaborate organizations to intercept plant shipments containing nematodes and other pests. Diseased and contaminated plant materials may be treated to kill the nematodes or their entry may be avoided. Quarantine also prevent the movement of infected plant and soil to move out to other nematodes free areas.

In USA, the soybean cyst nematode, *Heterodera glycines* has been subjected to Federal quarantine during 1954. State Quarantine was enforced against the potato cyst nematode, *Globodera rostochiensis* during the year 1941 in New York state. The burrowing nematode of citrus, *Radopholus similis* was brought under state Quarantine Act in Florida during 1953.

Plant Quarantine in India

The Destructive Insects and Pests Act, 1914 (DIP) was passed by the Government of India which restricts introduction of exotic pests and diseases into the country from abroad.

The Agricultural Pests and Disease Acts of the various states prevent interstate spread of pests within the country. The rules permits the Plant Protection Adviser to the Government of India or any authorised officer to undertake inspection and treatments.

Strict regulations have been made against *G. rostochiensis*, the potato cyst nematode and *Bursaphelenchus cocophilus*, the red ring nematode of coconut. Domestic quarantine regulations have also been imposed to restrict the movement of potato both for seed and table purposes in order to prevent the spread of potato cyst nematode from Tamil Nadu to other states in India.

Prevention of nematode spread

Nematodes do not move more than few centimetres a year on their own accord and most of them spread by passive means.

Nematodes spread mainly through air, soil, seed and water.

Heterodera cysts being very light in weight can be easily shifted to distant places in wind currents. This type of spread is common in sandy soil areas where dust storms facilitate this type of spread.

Soil adhering to potato tubers serves as a main source when such tubers are used as seed material. Besides labour, farm animals and farm implements also carry some amount of soil from nematode infested to a non-infested area.

Anguina tritici responsible for ear cockle disease of wheat is known to spread along with wheat seeds. Onion and lucerne bulbs spreads the stem and bulb nematode, *Ditylenchus dipsaci* from one place to another.

Movement of irrigation water and floods due to severe rain aids in the passive dispersal of the nematodes from one place to another.

Under the above circumstances, the following steps are to be taken.

Only nematode free seeds or seed materials should be used for raising crops.

The seed should be sown on land where nematode is not known to exist. If present, take some control measure and raise the crop.

The crops should be frequently inspected for the presence of the nematode.

Seed borne nematodes can be controlled by fumigation with methyl bromide. Hot water treatment of bulbs and other planting materials can be effectively used to prevent the spread of the nematodes.

Prevention of nematode multiplication

- Nematode multiplication can be prevented by withdrawing cultivation in nematode infected patches and such patches can be used for construction of buildings.
- Nematode multiplication can also be prevented by temporarily stopping cultivation of susceptible host plants. Crop rotation can also be adopted to prevent nematode multiplication.
- Seed certification can be adopted. Plant propagation material that is certified to be nematode free alone should be used for raising crops. For example banana suckers free of nematodes, potato seed pieces free of cyst nematode, garlic cloves free of stem nematode and wheat seeds free of seed galls can be produced commercially.
- Though the regulatory control has its own failures and shortcomings, it has reduced the rate of nematode spread in the country.

2. Physical Control

It is very easy to kill the nematodes in laboratory by exposing the nematodes to heat, irradiation, osmotic pressure, etc. But it is extremely difficult to adopt these methods under field conditions. These physical treatment may be hazardous to plant or the men working with the treatments and the radiation treatments may have residual effects.

Heat

Heat treatment of soil

Sterilization of soil by allowing steam is a practice in soil used in greenhouse, seed beds and also for small area of cultivation. Insects, weed seeds, nematodes, bacteria and fungi are killed by steam sterilization. In such cases steam is introduced into the lower level of soil by means of perforated iron pipes burried in the soil. The soil surface needs to be covered during steaming operation. Plastic sheets are used for covering.

In the laboratory and for pot culture experiments autoclaves are used to sterilize the soil.

Hot water treatment of planting material

Hot water treatment is commonly used for controlling nematodes. Prior to planting the seed materials such as banana corms, onion bulbs, tubers, seeds and roots of seedlings. They can be dipped in hot water at 50-55°C for 10 min before planting.

Irradiation

Irradiation also kills the nematodes. Cyst of *G. rostochiensis* exposed to 20,000g contained only dead eggs and 40,000g exposure, the eggs lost their contents. *Ditylenchus myceliophagus* in mushroom compost exposed to γ rays between 48,000 to 96,000g inactivatied the nematodes. UV light also kills the nematodes. But these irradiation is not practically feasible under field conditions.

Osmotic pressure

Feder (1960) reported 100% nematode mortality when sucrose or dextrose were added to nematode infested soil @ 1 to 5% by weight. But these methods are not practical and economical.

Washing process

Plant parasitic nematodes are often spread by soil adhering to potato tubers, bulbs and other planting materials. Careful washing of such planting material helps to avoid the nematodes spread into new planting field. Washing apparatus for cleaning potato and sugerbeet tubers are commercially developed and are being used in many countries.

Seed cleaning

Modern mechanical seed cleaning methods have been developed to remove the seed galls from normal healthy wheat seeds.

Ultrasonics

Ultrasonics have little effect on *Heterodera* spp. The use of this ultrasonics is not practically feasible.

3. Cultural Control

Cultural control methods are agronomical paractices employed in order to minimise nematode problem in the crops.

Selection of healthy seed material

In plants, propagated by vegetative means we can eliminate nematodes by selecting the vegetative part from healthy plants. The cyst nematodes of potato and the burrowing, spiral and lesion nematodes of banana can be eleminated by selecting nematode free planting materials. The wheat seed gall nematode and rice white tip nematode can be controlled by using nematode free seeds.

Adjusting the time of planting

Nematode life cycle depends on the climatic factors. Adjusting the time of planting helps to avoid nematode damage. In some cases, crops may be planted in winter when soil temperature is low and at that time the nematodes cannot be active at low temperature. Early potatoes and sugarbeets grown in soil during cold season and escapes cyst nematode damage since the nematodes are not that much active to cause damage to the crop during cold season.

Fallowing

Leaving the field without cultivation preferably after ploughing helps to expose the nematodes to sunlight and the nematodes die due to starvation without host plant. This method is not economical.

Deep summer ploughing

During the onset of summer, the infested field is ploughed with disc plough and exposed to hot sun, which inturn enhances the soil temperature and kills the nematodes.

For raising small nursery beds for vegetable crops like tomato and brinjal seed beds can be prepared during summer and covered with polythene sheets which enhances soil temperature by 5 to 10°C and thereby kills the nematodes in the seed bed. This method is very effective and nematode free seedlings can be raised by soil solarisation using polythene sheets.

Manuring

Raising green manure crops and addition of more amount of farm yard manure, oil cakes of neem and castor, pressmud, poultry manure, etc. enriches the soil and further encourages the development of predacious nematodes like

Mononchus spp. and also other nematode antagonistic microbes in the soil which checks the parasitic nematodes in the field.

Flooding

Flooding can be adopted where there is an enormous availability of water. Under submerged conditions, anaerobic condition develops in the soil which kills the nematodes by asphyxiation. Chemicals lethal to nematodes such as hydrogen sulphide and ammonia are released in flooded condition which kills the nematodes.

Trap cropping

Two crops are grown in the field, out of which one crops is highly susceptible to the nematode. The nematode attacks the susceptible crop. By careful planning, the susceptible crop can be grown first and then removed and burnt. Thus the main crop escapes from the nematode damage. Cowpea, a highly susceptible crop can be grown first and then removed and burnt. Cowpea is highly susceptible to root-knot nematode and the crop can be destroyed before the nematodes mature.

Antagonistic crops

Certain crops like mustard, marigold, neem, etc. have chemicals or alkaloids as root exudates which repel or suppress the plant parasitic nematodes.

In marigold (*Tagetes* spp.) plants, the alpha- terthinyl and biethinyl compounds are present throughout the plant from root to shoot tips. This chemicals kills the nematodes.

In mustard allyl isothiocyanate and in pangola grass pyrocatechol are present which kills the nematodes.

Such enemy plants can be grown along with main crop or included in crop rotation.

Removal and destruction of infected plants

Early detection of infested plants and their removal helps to reduce nematode spread. After harvest the stubbles of infested plants are to be removed. In tobacco, the root system is left in the field after harvest. This will serve as an inoculum for the next season crop. Similarly in *D. angustus* the nematode remains in the left out stubbles in the field after harvest of rice grains. Such stubbles are to be removed and destroyed and land needs to be ploughed to expose the soil.

Use of resistant varieties

Nematode resistant varieties have been reported from time to time in different crops. Use of resistant varieties is a very effective method to avoid nematode damage. **Nemared, Nematex, Hisar Lalit** and **Atkinson** are tomato varieties resistant to *M. incognita*. The potato variety **Kufri swarna** in resistant to *G. rostochiensis*.

4. Biological Control

Biological control aims to manipulate the parasites, predators and pathogens of nematodes in the rhizosphere in order to control the plant parasitic nematodes. Addition of organic amendments such as farm yard manure, oil cakes, green manure, pressmud, etc. encourages the multiplication of nematode antogonistic microbes which inturn checks the plant parasitic nematodes.

The addition of organic amendments acts in several ways against the plant parasitic nematodes. Organic acids such as formic, acetic, propionic and butyric acids are released in soil during microbial decomposition of organic amendments. Ammonia and hydrogen sulphide gases are also released in soil during decomposition. These organic acids and gases are toxic to nematodes.

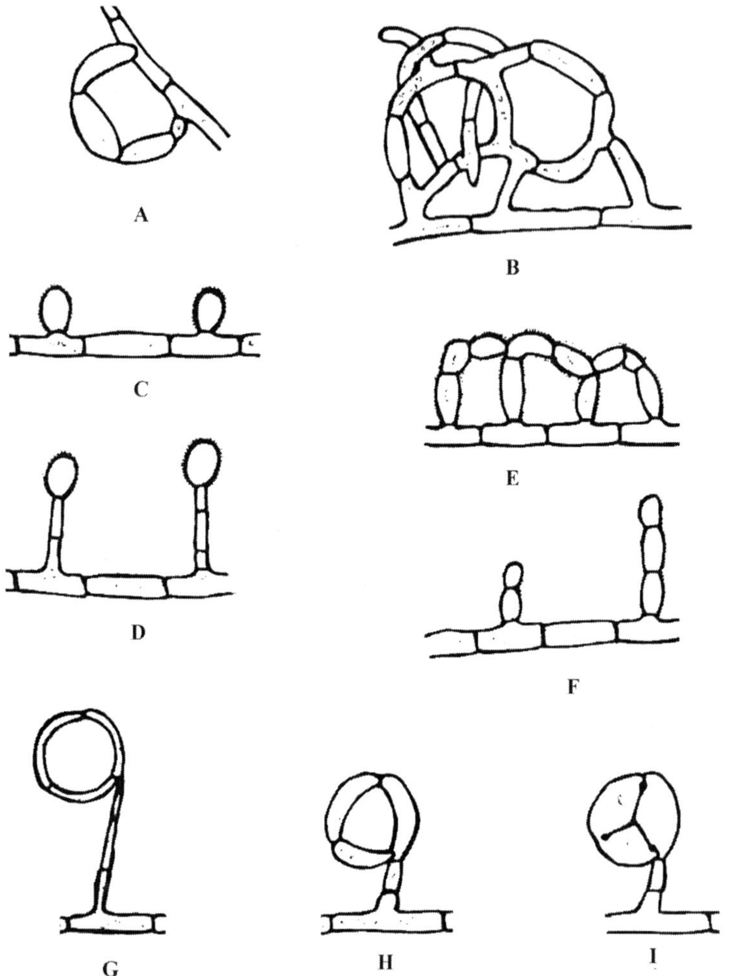

A. Simple ring **B.** Adhesive complex **C.** Three-dimensional traps; sessile **D.** Stalked **E.** Adhesive knobs and adhesive **F.** Simple two dimensional branches adhesive networks **G.** Non-constricting rings **H.** Constricting rings open **I.** Closed

Fig 19: Trapping organs of predatory nematophagous fungi

Nematode antagonistic microbes multiply rapidly due to addition of organic matter.

Organic amendments improve soil conditions and helps the plants to grow. The organic matter also provides nutrition for the crops plants.

Predacious nematodes

Predacious nematodes have specialised open stoma armed with teeth to catch and swallow the plant parasitic nematodes. Addition of organic amendments help to encourage the multiplication of predacious nematodes such as *Mononchus* spp. Other genera like *Diplogaster* spp. and *Tripyla* spp. also come under the group of predacious nematodes.

Predacious fungi

Most of the predacious fungi come under the order Moniliales and Phycomycetes. There are two types of predacious activities among these fungi. They are nematode trapping fungi and endozoic fungi.

Nematode Trapping Fungi (NTF)

The nematode trapping fungi have adhesive networks and sticky knobs are produced by the mycelium to capture the plant parasitic nematodes. The nematode trappers are grouped as follows.

Sticky branches: The fungal mycelia have short lateral branches and they anastamose to form loops. The nematodes are trapped in this loops.

Sticky networks: The mycelium curl around and anastamoses with similar branches. These loops produce complex three dimensional structures (Fig. 19A). The adhesive surface of the network helps to hold the nematode eg: *Arthrobotrys* spp. (Fig. 19 B).

Sticky knobs: Small spherical or subspherical lobes are present on one or two celled lateral hyphae. Only the terminal knob is sticky to hold the nematodes eg: *Monacrosporium ellipsospora.*

Constricting rings: The short hyphal branch curls back on itself and anastamoses and forming a ring. When the nematode enters the ring and contact the inner walls of the ring cells, the ring cells bulge inward filling the lumen of the ring and kills the nematode eg: *M. bombicoides* and *Dactylaria brochopaga.*

Non-constricting rings: The trap is formed similar to the constricting ring. It is a non-adhesive trap. The ring becomes an infective structure and kills the nematode eg: *Dactylaria candida.*

In addition to formation of traps and adhesive secretions, the predacious fungi may also produce toxin which kills the nematodes.

Endozoic fungi

The endozoic fungi usually enter the nematode by a germ tube that penetrates the cuticle from a sticky spore. The fungal hyphae ramify throughout the nematode body, absorb the contents and multiply. The hyphae then emerge from dead nematode. *Catenaria vermicola* often attacks sugarcane nematodes.

Parasitic fungi

Paecilomyces lilacinus is an effective egg parasite on many nematodes. The parasitic fungus is particularly effective against *Meloidogyne, Heterodera, Rotylenchulus* and *Tylenchulus.* The fungus attack the eggs as they are deposited in groups as a mass. The parasitic fungus was found to be effective against potato cyst nematode, root-knot nematodes in tomato, brinjal, betelvine and banana and *T. semipenetrans* in citrus.

Antagonistic fungi

Trichoderma spp. are one among a group of beneficial fungi that are present in almost all soils and diverse habitats. They have proven commercially viable as a successful biological control agent against plant parasitic nematodes and pathogenic fungi. Many species of *Trichoderma viz., T. viride, T. harzianum, T. koningi, T. longibrachiatum* and *T. hamatum* were reported effective against several nematodes.

Mechanism of action against phytonematodes

Mycoparasitism

Trichoderma spp. were reported to secrete many lytic enzymes like chitinase which help parasitism of *Meloidogyne* and *Globodera* eggs

Antibiosis

T. viride produces antibiotics like trichodermim, dermadin, trichoviridin and sesquiterpene heptalic acid which are involved in the suppression of pathogenic fungi and nematodes.

Competition

Competition for space or nutrients is one of the classical mechanisms of *Trichoderma* spp. They have high rhizosphere competency and can easily colonize the roots. This may reduce the feeding sites for nematodes.

Solubilization and sequestration of inorganic plant nutrients

Treatment with *T. harzianum* increased nitrogen uptake and also solubilized rock phosphate, Zn metal, Mn^{4+}, Fe^{3+} and Cu^{2+}. Enhanced nutrient uptake increases the tolerance of the plants to nematode attack.

Induced Systemic Resistance

Defense enzymes *viz.,* peroxidase, polyphenoloxidase, phenylalanine ammonia lyase, catalase and chitinase were induced more in *T. viride* treated plants which determine the ability of the plant to survive any nematode attack.

Bacteria

Plant growth promoting rhizobacteria for nematode management

Bacteria that colonize the rhizosphere soil under the chemical influence of the root are commonly referred to as rhizobacteria. Specific rhizobacteria that have the ability to improve plant growth are called as plant growth promoting rhizobacteria (PGPR)

Species of rhizobacteria used for nematode management

Agrobacterium sp	*Burkholderia* sp
Arthrobacterium sp	*Azospirillum* sp
Azotobacter sp	*Bacillus* sp
Clostridium sp	*Chromobacterium* sp
Disulfovibrio sp	*Corynebacterium* sp
Serratia	*Pseudomonas* sp

Mechanism of action of PGPR

a) Antibiotic-Mediated Suppression: Antibiotic production is one of the main mechanisms involved in the suppression of plant pathogens which includes both nematodes and pathogens by fluorescent pseudomonads. Antibiotics include phenazines, tropolone, pyrrolnitrin, pyocyanin and 2,4- diacetylphloroglucinol.

b) Siderophore-Mediated Suppression: Pseudomanas fluorescens generally produce yellow green, water soluble, fluorescent siderophores which are linked with their disease suppression ability. This efficient iron uptake mechanism helps these strains to aggressively colonize plant roots thus aiding the physical displacement of deleterious organisms.

c) Induced Systemic Resistance: Induced Systemic Resistance (ISR) is based on plant defence mechanisms that are activated by inducing agents. ISR once expressed activates multiple potential defence mechanisms viz., increased activity of chitinases, peroxidases and other pathogenesis-related proteins, accumulation of phytoalexins and formation of protective biopolymers, e.g. lignin, callose and hydroxyproline-rich glycoproteins.

Pasteuria

Pasteuria penetrans was found to be very effective against the root-knot nematodes in many crops. The *P. penetrans* infested J_2 of root-knot nematodes can be seen attached with spores throughout the cuticle (Plate 18).

The life cycle of *Pasteuria penetrans* consists of four stages: spore germination, vegetative growth, fragmentation and sporogenesis. The electrostatic forces on the spores help attach themselves to the nematode cuticle in the soil. Such attached spores germinate by forming a germ tube and penetrate into the nematode cuticle in about 3 days after infection. The bacterial thalli then start spreading and form spherical **microcolony** or **mother colony** with dichotomously branched mycelium in about 14 days after infection. Four celled stage of the bacterium, called **quartet**, is observed in about 18 days after infection. Later quartets fragment into 2 celled stage called **doublets** which develop into unicellular stage on the 24th day by further fragmentation. Mature spores of the bacterium are formed in about 30 days after infection synchronizing with the life cycle of the host nematode (Fig. 20).

5. Chemical Control

The term pesticide is used to those chemicals which are highly poisonous and control the animal and plant species. Chemicals which kill the nematodes are called nematicides. Nematicide is defined as a substance or mixture of substances used for killing, repelling or otherwise preventing the plant parasitic nematodes. A chemical may be called as repellent if it prevents the pest species from attacking its host and an attractant, if the pest species is attracted to the source, trapped and killed.

The primary advantage of chemical control over the other methods is that the pest population is brought under control within a shorter period of time due to quick knockdown effect on the target organisms. This is the reason that the growers tend to employ chemical control quite often than that of other methods. Many nematode species attack the crop plants during the seedling stage and cause severe damage to the root. Seedlings raised from nematicide treated beds are usually healthy with good root system. Another important benefit resulting from chemical treatment is that in addition to nematodes, fungi, bacteria and weeds are also controlled. Damage caused by nematodes could not be fully appreciated until chemical nematicides were applied to soil in many parts of the world resulting in dramatic improvement in the crop growth. Plant parasitic nematodes can be controlled by applying nematicides to the soil or on the host plant. Spot application of nematicides is the efficient and economic method, since it requires less active ingredient and avoids the need to treat the great bulk of soil in which the crop will be grown or already growing. The nematicides should be applied only on need based and their use can improve the plant growth and yield.

History of chemical control

Kuhn (1881) first tested CS_2 to control sugarbest nematode in Germany and he could not get encouraging results. In south Carolina State, U.S.A, Bessey (1911) treated CS_2 for the control of root-knot nematodes but the method proved impractical. Later on the chemicals like formaldehyde, cyanide and quicklime were observed to have nematicidal properties, but all these chemicals were found to be highly expensive.

Mathews(1919) observed the effect of chloropicrin (tear gas) against plant parasitic nematodes in England. Carter (1943) an Entomologist of Hawaii, Pineapple Research Institute reported the efficacy of 1,3 dichloropropene 1,2 dichloropropane (DD) mixture @ 250 lb/acre, against the plant parasitic nematodes. In 1944, scientists from California and Florida states of USA reported the efficacy of ethylene dibromide (EDB). In the same year the Dow Chemical Company, USA introduced the chemical as a soil fumigant for the management of nematodes. The introduction of these two nematicides *viz.*, DD and EDB paved way for the chemical control of nematodes.

Classification of pesticides

The pesticides can be classified based on their mode of entry mode of action and also by their chemical nature.

Classification based on mode of entry

Stomach poison: The chemicals are applied on the foliage and other parts of plant when ingested by the nematode, it act on the digestive system and cause death. These types of chemicals should be palatable for the pest species and able to bring death quickly. The common examples are Lead Arsenate and Phosphomidon.

Contact poison: The toxicant which brings death of the pest species by means of contact and are directly absorbed by the cuticle. The chemical also penetrates into the body through the cuticle. e.g. Methyl parathion.

Fumigants: The toxicant in its gaseous state penetrates the organism and kills them. CS_2, DD and EDB are examples for fumigants.

Classification based on mode of action

Physical poison: The toxicant which brings death of an organism by exerting a physical effect is known as physical poison. The heavy oils like tar oil leads to asphyxiation and cause death. Chemicals like aluminium oxide abrade the cuticle and leads to loss of body moisture to kill nematodes.

Protoplasmic poison: A toxicant resposible for precipitation of protein, especially destruction of cellular protoplasm of intestinal epithelium. Heavy metals such as mercury and copper, fatty acids, formaldehyde, ethyleneoxide, nitrophenols, fluorine compounds and arsenic compounds come under this group.

Respiratory poison: A chemical which blocks cellular respiration or inactivate cellular respiratory enzymes are respiratory poisons. The chmicals such as H_2S, DD and EDB are examples of this group.

Nerve poison: These chemicals have anti acetylcholinesterase activity which leads to constant excitation of the nerves in the target organism. Due to this, the organism faces convulsions, tremors, muscle paralysis and leads to death. Diazinon and aldicarb are examples of nerve poison.

Classification based on chemical nature

Systemic inorganic compounds: These compounds are systemic inorganic salts which act as stomach poisons and kill the target organism. e.g. Copper aceto arsenate and calcium arsenate.

Synthetic organic compounds: These group are further classified as

Halogenated hydrocarbon: e.g. Chloropicrin, methyl bromide, DD, EDB and DBCP.

Organophosphorus compounds: The basic constituents of organophosphorus compound are carbon, hydrogen and chlorine and certain compounds may have oxygen and sulphur also. e.g. Parathion, Dichlofenthion, Thionazin, Fenamiphos, Fensulphothion, Ethoprop and Phorate

Carbamates: Carbamate compounds are derivatives of carbamic acid. The key feature for their nematicidal activity is their structural resemblance to acetylcholine and thus have affinity for enzyme cholinesterase. Further, the structure has a bulky side chain capable of interacting with the anionic site of cholinesterase. Carbamates are reversible cholinesterase inhibitors and highly cholinergic as that of organophosphorus compounds. Poisoned organisms show violent convulsions and other neuromuscular disturbances due to inhibition of cholinesterase. Metham sodium, aldicarb, carbofuran, etc.are examples of carbamates.

Substituted phenols: In these compounds the phenol is substituted by any other group e.g. Binapacryl.

Thiocyanates: e.g. Lethane and Thanite.

Fluorine compounds: Fluorine sodium fluoroacetate.

Sulphur compounds: e.g. CS_2, H_2S and Endosulfan.

Natural products

The natural products include compounds like nicotine, pyrethrin, oil cakes of neem, castor, pungam, ect. The chemical alpha terthinyl compounds found in marigold plants have excellent nematicidal property. Catechol in root diffusate of *Ergrostis curvula* is highly toxic to *Meloidogyne* populations.

Pesticide formulation

It is essential that the toxicant must be amenable for application in an effective manner so as to come into direct contact with the target organism or leave an uniform and persistent deposit upon the plant surface. Only a small quantity of the toxicant is required to be distributed over a large area and rarely the toxicant is to be made available in a diluted form or in a form easily distributed. Thus the toxicants are combined with carriers, diluents and surface active agents to ensure uniform distribution of small quantity of pesticide over large area to minimise the use of chemical and to avoid phytotoxicity. The chemical can be obtained in required concentration diluting them with water and their action can be improved by incorporating them with activated synergists, adhesives, attractants and repellants.

Different pesticide formulations are as follows

Dusts: In a dust formulation the toxicant is diluted either by mixing with or by impregnation on a suitably finely divided carrier. The carrier may be an organic flour or pulverised mineral or clay. The toxicant in a dust formulation ranges from 0.65 to 25 per cent. Dusts are defined as those having a particle size less than 100 micron and with decrease in particle size the toxicity of the formulation increases. The dust should flow freely and must not cake or ball in the hopper. Dust application must be done in a calm weather and early in the morning when the plant is wet with dew.

Wettable powder (WP): Wettable powder is a powdered formulation which yields stable suspension when diluted with water. The active ingredient in such formulation ranges from 15 to 95 per cent. e.g. *Aldoxicarb* 75 WP and carbofuran 50/75 WP.

Emulsifiable Concentrates (EC): This formulation contains the toxicant, a solvent for the toxicant and an emulsifying agent. It is a clear solution and yields an emulsion of oil in water when diluted with water. When sprayed the solvent evaporates quickly leaving a deposit of toxicant from which water also evaporates. e.g. Malathion 50 EC and Fenamiphos 40 EC.

Water Soluble Concentrates (WSC): These are liquid formulations and similar to wettable powders except in the type of formulation.

Granular formulations: They are used at 2-15 per cent concentration. The size of the granules varies between 30-60 micron. They can be applied in marshy areas and very easy to handle and apply in the field e.g. Carbofuran 3 G and Phorate 10 G.

Soluble powders: They are in powder form and soluble in water e.g. Acephate 75 SP.

Low volume concentrates: The technical grade of the toxicant is normally at highly concentrated level. They are dissolved in nonvolatile solvents. They are applied to plants with ultra low volume sprayers. e.g. Malathion 95 LVC and Dimecron 100 LVC.

Fumigants: Fumigants are employed to control great variety of pests *viz.,* pests of stored products, household articles, nematodes and other subterranean insects. DD, EDB and DBCP are some of the fumigants. They get converted into gas which is toxic to the nematodes.

Seed dressers: These chemicals can be in liquid or powder form for treating the seeds. Gum is usually added to the seed dressing chemical in order to stick with the seed coat. e.g. Carbofuran 40 F and Carbofuran 50 SD.

Types of chemical treatment

Preplant treatment: The halogenated hydrocarbons are highly phytotoxic and such chemicals should be apply in a nematode infested field or seed bed before raising the crop. A waiting period of 3 to 4 weeks must elapse between the application and planting or sowing. Normally fumigants are used as preplant treatment.

Treatment at planting: The chemicals which come under the group organophosphate and dithiocarbamates are comparatively less phytotoxic and such chemicals can be applied at the time of planting.

Post plant treatment: Post plant treatment is given after raising the crop. Normally it is advised to complete the nematicidal treatment within a month after planting or sowing in case of annual crops. In perennial crops like citrus, grapevine, etc. the nematicides are to be applied every year depending on the infestation level. Organophosphates and dithiocarbamates can be applied to the standing crop.

Bare root-dip treatment: Chemicals like monocrotophos and phosphamidon can be used for seedling root-dip treatment. The nematicide solutions are prepared by diluting with required amount of water and the seedling roots are dipped in the solution for 5 - 10 minutes and then planted in the field.

Seed treatment: In seed treatment, the chemicals are treated to the seeds along with sticking substances like gum in order to make a coat on the surface of the seed. A special formulation carbofuran 40 F are used as seed treatment in order to protect the plants from nematodes in early growth period.

Foliar treatment: The systemic and contact compounds can be sprayed on the foliage to control the aerial nematodes pests. The systemic compounds are absorbed and translocated throughout the plant including the root system due to basipetal action.

Types of Application

Broadcast: Application of nematicide over an entire area of the infested field. The method of applications used when crops are to be planted in rows with the spacing of 60 cm or below. Normally nematicide granules are applied by this broadcast method.

Row application: Here, the chemicals are applied along the plant rows thereby the quantity of nematicide is very much reduced than that of the broadcast method. This row application can be efficiently employed in crops grown in rows with the spacing of more than 60 cm. This type of application holds good for crops like cotton, tobacco, chilli and other vegetable crops.

Spot application: This is a commonly employed method for annual crops which are widely spaced. This method is very economical since the chemicals are applied to the rhizosphere.

Strip application: In this method the planting strip alone is treated with the chemical. This strip application holds good for some perennial crops like grapevine and citrus where 50 per cent of the chemical is saved than the broadcast application.

Site application: The site application is commonly employed for replant problems in established vineyards. It is also feasible with wide-spaced annual crops such as melons. For melons, a treating site of 60 sq.cm is sufficient while tree crops require a minimum area of 2 to 2.5m. The site application reduces the quantity of nematicides to be used to a considerable extent.

Description of some important nematicides

Ethylene dibromide (EDB): 1.2 - Dibromomethane. It is a colourless liquid and the gas is non-inflammable. It is available as 83% liquid formulation containing 1.2 kg active ingredient per litre and as 35% granules. It is injected or dibbled into the soil for the control of nematodes at 60 to 120 l or 200 kg a.i./ha but it is not very effective against cyst nematodes, *Heterodera* spp. and soil fungi. Crops like onion, garlic and other bulbs should not be planted after soil treatment with EDB. It is available as Bromofume and Dowfume.

Dibromochloropropane: (DBCP) 1,2-dibromo-3-chloro-propane. It is a straw coloured liquid, a litre of it weighing 1.7 kg. It can be used as soil treatment before planting, at the time of planting or as post plant treatment for the control of nematodes. The chemical is effective when the soil temperature is above 20°C. It is applied as a sprinkle and also mixed with irrigation water. Recommended @ 10-60 l/ha depending upon the crop and stage. Certain crops like tobacco and potato are sensitive due to high bromine content in the chemical. It functions more efficiently than other fumigants at high soil temperature due to its high boiling point (195.6^{o}C). Trade names are Nemagon and Fumazone.

D.D. mixture: It is the trade name of the mixture of compounds, chief of them contain the cis and the trans isomers in equal quantities of 1,3-dichloropropene 30.35%, and a few other chlorinated compounds up to about 5%. Of these, dichloropropene is the most toxic component and among its two isomers, the transisomer is twice as toxic as the cis-isomer. It is a black liquid of 100% formulation and a litre of it contains approximately 1 kg of technical compound. It is used in the control of soil insects and nematodes and injected into the soil at a depth of 15-20 cm at 25 x 30 cm spacing. It is a fungicide at very high doses. Since it is highly phytotoxic, it is used for preplant soil application at least 2-3 weeks before planting. It is used as such at 225-280 l/ ha, but in clay and peaty soils a higher dosage is required. It taints potato tubers and carrots grown in treated soil. Dichloropropene is available under the trade name Telone and in mixture with dibromoethane under the name Dorlone

Methylbromide or Bromomethane: It boils at 4.5°C. At ordinary temperatures it is a gas and therefore, confined in containers under pressure as a liquid. The gas is 1.5 times as heavy as air. Its insecticidal properties were described by Le Goupil in 1932. Its power of penetration into packed foodstuffs such as flour is remarkable. As it kills insects slowly a longer period of exposure to gas may be required. For control of stored grain pests it is used at 24-32 g/m^3, exposure period being 48 h. In tent fumigation for the control of termites and powder post beetles, the dosage recommended is 32-64 g/m^3. For fumigating live plants, the dosage is 16-32 g/m^3. Some plants are likely to be injured. In soil application for the control of nematodes and insects it is applied at 4.7 ml/sq.ft. It also kills insects, rodents fungi and weeds in the soil. It is highly dangerous cumulative poison to warm blooded animals. The technicians using the fumigant must always wear a gas mask. A halide detector lamp shows a blue flame if the gas is present. Addition of chloropicrin to cylinders containing methylbromide (commercial product Dowfume MC-2 contains 2% chloropicrin) is also done so that the gas when persists in an area causes irritation to eyes.

Chloropicrin or Trichlorodimethane: Trade names are: Acquinite and Picfume. It is the tear gas which is non-inflammable with good penetrating effect. It does not bleach or tarnish but corrodes metals slightly. It should not be used for fumigating germinated seeds or growing young plants. For the control of stored grain pests, it is recommended at 16-48 g/m^3. Being low volatile compound the gas persists for a longer period and its removal is rather difficult.It is useful in the control of nematodes and insects in the soil.

Fensulfothion: C_{11} H_{17} O_1 PS_2; 1,1-diethyl 1-0-p (methyl sulfinyl) phenyl phosphonate. Trade names are Dassanit and Terracur. It is a systemic nematicide and has long persistence. It has been found effective against golden nematode of potatoes in the Nilgiris. The chemical is also effective against turf nematodes.

Fenamiphos: $C_{13}H_{22}$ No3 PS; 0-ethyl-0 (methyl1-4-ethylthiophenyl) is opropylamidophosphate. Trade name Nemacur. It is a systemic nematicide used for the control of root-knot and cyst forming nematodes. It is available as 5 or 10% granule. It is also available as 40 EC. When applied on the foliage it brings about death of the nematodes in the roots as the toxicant gets translocated basipetally to the roots. LD_{50} for male rate: oral 15.3; dermal 500.

Ethoprop: 0-ethyl S, S-dipropyl phosphoraodithioate. Its trade name is Mocap. It is available as 10% granule. It is a non systemic nematicide with very little persistence. The chemical is very effective when the juvenile nematodes are at peak population in the soil.

Phorate: 0,0-diethyl S-(ethylthiomethyl) phosphorodithioate. Trade name is Thimet. It is a systemic insecticide cum nematicide, available as 10% granule. It has got both contact and fumigant action. It does not persist for a longer period and gets metabolically oxidised yielding phosphorothioate and sulfone, which are readily hydrolysed. LD_{50} for rat: oral 16 to 3.7; dermal 2.5 to 6.2.

Metham sodium: Sodium N-methyldithio carbamate. It is available in the trade names as Vapam, Sistan, Vitafume and Unifume. It is recommended at a dose of 100-200 ml/m^2. The solution is readily mixed with water and can be applied as soil drench or injected into the soil. The chemical after treatment produces a gas and distribution through the soil may result from dispersion in water or gaseous diffusion. It is used as a preplanting treatment and effective against insects, fungi, nematodes, weeds and other pests. It is highly phytotoxic and a waiting period of 2 weeks need to be allowed between application and planting.

Aldicarb:2-methyl-2 (methylthio) propionaldehyde O (methylcarbomyl) oxime. Trade name is Temik. The sulphur atom in the molecule is oxidised to sulfoxide and then to sulfone. It is a systemic 10% granule. The residues remain in plants for 30-35 days as a lethal dose. It also acts as repellant, contact nematicide and interferes with reproduction of the nematodes by way of sex reversal.

Carbofuran: C_{12} H_{15} No_3. It is 2,3-dihydro-2, 2-dimethyl 7 benzofuranyl methyl carbamate. Trade name Furadan. It is a systemic insecticide cum nematicide. It is formulated as 3% granule and also as 40 F. The residual effect lasts for 30-60 days. It has also got phytotonic effect. This systemic chemical has got acropetal action and applied @ 1-2 kg a.i/ha.

Methomyl: S-methyl thiomethyl carbamoyl thioacetamidate. It is effective against insects, mites and nematodes. The trade name is Lannate.

Oxamyl: Methyl N, N-dimethyl - N (methylcarbamoyloxy) - 1 thiooxamidate. It is formulated as 40 EC. It is a systemic chemical. It is effective against the foliar nematodes and can be sprayed on the foliage. Trade name Vydate.

Care while handling pesticides

Pesticides being toxic to human beings and domestic animals should be handled with utmost care. The following precautions should always be observed.

- The pesticids should always be stored in their original containers and kept in a locked cupboard where they are out of reach of the children and domestic animals.

- They should be kept away from food or foods stuffs and medicines.
- The instruction found on the labels should be carefully read and strictly followed.
- Bags and containers of pesticides should be cut open with a separate knife intended for such purposes.
- The empty containers after using the chemical should be destroyed and should not be put into some other use.
- While preparing the spray solutions bare hands should not be used for mixing the chemical with water.
- Inhaling of pesticide sprays, dusts, smoking, chewing, eating or drinking while mixing or applying the chemicals should be avoided.
- As far as possible spilling of pesticides on slin or clothing should be avoided. The clothes should be washed after each operation.
- Particles or drops of pesticides which may accidentally get into eyes should be flushed out immediately with large volumes of clean water.
- It is preferable that protective clothing and devices are used while handling poisonous chemicals to avoid exposure to sprays or drifts.
- Dusting or spraying should never be done against the wind and it is preferable to have them done in cool and calm weather.
- While spraying, sprayer nozzles if get blocked should not be blown by mouth. Washers and other contaminated parts should be buried.
- After handling pesticides, hands, face and body should be washed and clothing changed.
- Washing of equipment after use and containers in or near wells or streams shoul be avoided.
- Persons engaged in handling pesticides should undergo regular medical check up.
- In case of any suspected poisoning due to insecticides the nearest physician should be called on immediately.

First Aid Precautions

Swallowed poisons: Remove poison from the patient's stomach immediately by inducing vomiting. Give common salt 15g in a glass of warm water and emetic and repeat until vomit fluid is clear. Gently touching the throat with the finger induce vomiting when the stomach is full of fluid. If the patient is already vomiting do not give emetic and give large amount of water.

Inhaled poison: Carry the patient to fresh air immediately. Open all the doors and windows to provide sufficient fresh air. Loosen all tight clothing. Provide artificial respiration, if breathing has stopped or irregular. It the patient is convulsing, keep him in bed in some dark room.

Skin contamination: Wash the skin with excess water several times.

Eye contamination: Hold the eyelids open. Wash the eyes gently with water immediately. Give several such washings until physician arrives.

Antidotes

Removal of poison: Remove poison by inducing vomiting and the universal antitode which is the mixture of 7g of activated charcoal, 3.5g of magnesium oxide and 3.5g tannic acid in half a glass of warm water may be used to absorb or neutralize poisons. This mixture is useful in poisoning by acids, liquid gylcosides and heavy metals.

16

Entomophilic Nematodes

Nematode associated with insects are referred as entomophilic, entomogenous and entomophagous nematodes. Generally they belong to the superfamilies Tylenchoidea, Rhadbitoidea, Oxyuroidea and Mermithoidea of the phylum Nematoda.

Nature of parasitism

Christie (1914) divided the nematodes associated with invertebrates into three groups.

- Those nematodes which live in the alimentary tract of he invertebrates.
- Those nematodes which are more or less closely related to free living species and often have a combination of saprophagous and parasitic habits.
- Those nematodes which parasitizes the body cavity or tissue of their host.

Entomophilic nematodes are group of parasites that cause debilitation, sterility or death of insects. Entomophilic nematodes vary greatly in size and shape having the insects as intermediate or as definite hosts. Many group of insects are parasitised by nematodes.

The earliest known nematode parasite of insect is *Mermis nigrescens* from grass hopper. *M. nigrescens* is a common parasite on grass hopper, locusts and also on other insects.These insects become infested with *M. nigrescens* by feeding on vegetation where the dark brown nematode eggs are deposited. These hosts are vulnerable to infection by nematode through their life cyle. Developing female nematode remain longer in the host and directly proportional to the size of the host. *M. nigrescens* parasites on *Schistocerca gregaria* and the other parasitic nematodes on grass hopper include *Agamermis decaudata* and *Hexamermis albicans.*

The developing *M. nigrescens* affects the morphology and physiology of host insect. They also affect host mobility and host size. The gut and oviducts become compressed and distorted. Cuticle become discoloured and softened.

Sterilisation of female host, inhibition of moulting, reduced excretion is also observed. The mermithid parasitism is always fatal to the host.

The mermithid nematode, *Romanomermis culicivorax* has been successfully mass produced for commercial preparation as a biological control agent against mosquitoes. Mermithids that develop in the larval host are always lethal to their host. The aquatic habit allows this nematode to reach high levels of parasitism. It kills mosquito before it pupates which eliminates the adult stage of the insect. It is commercially marketed as "**Skeeter Doom**".

The nematode, *Leidynema appendicullata* has been reported to infect the rectum of the cockroach, *Gromphadorhina portentosa. Periplaneta americana* is infected with *Hammerschmidtiella diesingi.*

The nematode, *Cephalonbium microbivorum* was recorded from the hindgut of criket, *Gryllus assimilis*. The intestine of *G. domesticus* being affected by the nematode, *Protiellatus alii* and only one female was found in each host. The intestine and oesophagus of the mantids, *Polyspilota aeruginosa* and *Mantis viridis* are infected by the nematode, *Gynopceilla pseudovipara.*

The juvenile nematode, *Parasitohabdites piniperdae* are found in the larval haemocoel of the bark beetle, *Myleophilus piniperda*. The nematode, *Sulphuretylenchus elongatus* can directly penetrate and kill about 8% of eggs and 2-4% larval stage of the fir engraver, *Scolytus ventralis*. The nematode infection also delays the emergence of adults,reduces the longevity, affect reproductive organs and reduce the fecundity.

The nematode, *Sphaerulariopsis dendroctoni* is an obligate parasite and does not kill its bark beetle host, *Denroctonus retipennis*. The Ips *confusus* infected with *Contorylenchus elongatus* has reduced brood emergence and fertility.

The nematode, *Sphaerularia bomi* is associated with bumble bees. *S. bombi* parasitism sterilizes the queen, the flight of queen was unsteady, inhabit the development of ovaries and are also reduced to translucent filaments.

Entomopathogenic nematodes

In the recent years, a new interest has been kindled on the entomopathogenic nematodes belonging to the families Steinernematidae and Heterorhabditidae due to their excellent potential and quick knock down effect on insects. Research on biological control of insects with entomopathogenic nematodes has progressed since 1932, with the discovery of *Steinernema glaseri* infecting the Japanese beetle.

Entomopathogenic nematodes are mutually symbiotic with the bacteria *Xenorhabdus*. and *Photorhabdus* spp. and these bacteria are responsible for the death of the host. The bacteria are gram negative, non spore forming, rod shaped and facultatively anaerobic. They occur as primary and secondary forms and the primary forms produce a wide spectrum of antibiotics.

The third stage dauer juveniles (DJ_3) of these nematodes are the only stages outside the host and resistant to environmental stress. The DJ3 enter through the natural openings of the host as mouth and anus. On entering the host, they reach the haemocoel and release the bacteria from their intestine, which multiply and suppress the immunity of the host by causing the disease **septicaemia.** Consequently, the host is killed within 48 hrs. In turn, the entomopathogenic nematodes feed upon the bacteria and host tissues, pass 1 to 2 generations, multiply 10^5 times and leave the host as DJ_3.

Entomopathogenic nematodes are highly potential biocontrol agents for several lepidopteran and coleopteran insect pests. The desirable attributes of entomopathogenic nematodes like their wide spectrum activity, ability to kill their hosts within short periods, efficient mass culturing techniques and exemption by the Environmental Protection Agency for registration have stimulated strong commercial interest as biological agent that can be incorporated into pest management practices. A number of commercial products containing entomopathogenic nematodes are available in the world market namely ORTHO Biosafe, X-GNAT, Magnet, Nemasys, Entonem, Otinem, etc.

Phoretic relation

The nematodes are carried from gallery to gallery and from tree to tree externally on various parts of the insects such as beneath the elytra, between intersegmentel folds, on tarsal and tibial joints of the legs and internally in the gut, malpighian tubules, reproductive system and trachea. After being transported to a new environment the nematodes feed on microorganisms in the beetle's galleries. The phoretic nematodes have adopted to their host so that only a certain stage is transported to a new environment. The stage is often a resistant form known as dauer juvenile or dauer larva.

The dauer juveniles can be found under the oily cuticle of elytra and between thoracic folds. Often the juveniles are arranged in series with one another or occur in clumps or bundles. The oily cucticle provides adhesive substance and protects nematodes from desiccation. The dauer juveniles of *Goodeys* spp. are found under the elytra of female, *Scolytus scolytus.*

The wilt disease of pine tree is caused by pine wood nematode, *Bursaphelenchus xylophilus*. The Cerambycidae beetle, *Monochamus alternatus* carries the nematodes as vector. Dauer larvae enter through abdominal spiracles. The nematode are also found on the body surface, the abdomen and the tail tip.

Important entomophilic nematodes recorded in India.

Name of the nematode	Host	Reference
Neotylenchus sp.	*Scirpophaga nivella*	David (1962)
Panagrolaimus sp.	*Chilo zonellus*	Mathur *et al.* (1966)
Rhabditis sp.	*Chilo zonellus*	
Pelodera rhychophori	*Rhyncophorus ferrugineus*	Muthukrishnan (1971)
Mermithids	*Parallelia algira*	Hussian & Khan (1966)
Mermithids	*Sogota pallascens*	Purohit *et al.* (1967)
Mermis sp.	*Amsacto moorei*, *Cirphis* sp.	Bindra & Kittur (1956)
Mermis sp.	*Epilema* sp.	Mathur (1959)
		Argyroploce cellifera
Mermis sp.	*Anomis flava,*	
	Sylepta balteata,	
	Hyblaea puera	
Agamermis sp.	*Trypozyza incertulas*	Rao (1958)
Hexamermis sp.	*Chilo infuscatellus,*	Srivastava (1964)
	C. auricillia	
	Scirpophaga nivella	
Hexamermis sp.	*Spodoptera maurita*	Murad (1969)
Leidynema	*Blatta orientalis appendiculata*	Rao (1958)
Psilocephala	*Gryllotalpa afticana*	Rao (1958)
Singhiella singhi	*G. africana*	Rao (1958)
Binema sp.	*G. africana*	Basir (1956)
Talpicola arnata	*G. africana*	Basir (1956)
T. mirzaia	*G. africana*	Basir (1956)
Cameronia biovata	*G. africana*	Basir (1948)
Protellus indicus	*P. humberteana*	Muthukrishnan (1971)
Neoplantine	*P. humberteana monospinosus*	Muthukrishnan (1971)
Agalpterixia	*P. humberteana coimbatorensis*	Muthukrishnan (1971)
Crydiella corydi	*Corydiana petriveniana*	Rao & Rao (1956)
Blatticola blatticola	*Blata germinica*	Basir (1940)
B. superllaimi	*Supella supellitillum*	Rao & Rao (1956)
Psuedonymus klossi	*Dytiscus marginalis*	Farooqui (1967)
P. mehdi	*D. marginalis*	Farooqui (1967)
Thelastoma alighori	*P. americana*	Basir (1942)
T. indiana	*P. lucophae*	Basir (1942)

17

Caenorhabditis Elegans as a Biological Model System

Model organisms are widely used in biological researches to describe basic biological processes. When selecting living organisms as models to work with, a wide range of characteristics are used which include: 1) rapid development with short life cycles, 2) small adult size, 3) ready availability and 4) tractability. Being small, growing rapidly and being readily available are crucial in terms of housing them, given the budget and space limitations of research and teaching laboratories. Tractability relates to the ease with which they can be manipulated. Many model organisms have been used including fruit fly, *Drosophila melanogaster*, the most obvious organism used for teaching Mendelian genetics and developmental biology; *Escherichia coli*, a favoured organism for molecular biological studies involving recombinant DNA technology. Research into the molecular and developmental biology of *C. elegans* was begun in 1974 by Sydney Brenner and it has since been used extensively as a model organism.

C. elegans is a popular research organism as it possesses all the characteristics mentioned, yet shares many essential biological properties with humans. For instance, researchers who study apoptosis (programmed cell death) use *C. elegans* as an experimental organism in the hope of finding treatments for certain types of human cancers, such as leukaemia.

C. elegans is easy and inexpensive to maintain in laboratory conditions with a diet of *E. coli*. Embryogenesis occurs in about 12 hours, development to the adult stage occurs in 2.5 days and the life span is 2-3 weeks. The short, hermaphroditic life cycle (~3 days) and large number (300+) of offspring of *C. elegans* allows large-scale production of animals within a short period of time. Since *C. elegans* has a small body size, *in vivo* assays can be conducted in a 96 well microplate. Laboratory stocks of *C. elegans* can even be stored in liquid nitrogen for 25 years without losing their viability. The transparent body allows clear observation of all cells in mature and developing animals. Furthermore, the intensively studied genome, complete cell lineage map, knockout (KO) mutant libraries and established genetic methodologies including mutagenesis, transgenesis and RNA interference (RNAi) provide a variety of options to manipulate and study *C. elegans* at the molecular level and for a more detailed presentation of genetic and genomic resources.

The *C. elegans* genome size is relatively small (9.7×10^7 base pairs or 97 Megabases), when compared to the human genome which is estimated to consist of 3 billion base pairs (3×10^9 bp or 3000 Megabases). The entire *C. elegans* genome has been sequenced. Several novel molecular biological techniques exist for *C. elegans* can be used by researchers for studying higher eukaryotes. **Fig. 19:** Anatomy of *C. elegans* (hermaphrodite)

In 2002, the Nobel Prize in Physiology or Medicine was awarded to Sydney Brenner, H. Robert Horvitz and John Sulston for their work on the genetics of organ development and programmed cell death (PCD) in *C. elegans*. The 2006 Nobel Prize in Physiology or Medicine was awarded to Andrew Fire and Craig C. Mello, for their discovery of RNA interference in *C. elegans.* In 2008 Martin Chalfie shared a Nobel Prize in Chemistry for his work on green fluorescent protein (GFP) in *C. elegans*.

Because all research into *C. elegans* essentially started with Sydney Brenner in the 1970s, many scientists either worked as a post-doctoral or post-graduate researcher in Brenner's lab or in the lab of someone who previously worked with Brenner went on to establish their own worm research labs. Where there is a fairly well documented 'lineage' of *C. elegans* scientists. This lineage was recorded in some detail at the 2003 International Worm Meeting and the results were stored in the Wormbase database.

C. elegans made news when it was discovered that specimens had survived the Space Shuttle *Columbia* disaster in February 2003. Later, in January 2009, live samples of *C. elegans* from the University of Nottingham spent two weeks on the International Space Station as part of a project to explore the effects of zero gravity on muscle development and its physiology.

General Biology of *C. elegans*

C. elegans is a saprophytic nematode species that has often been described as inhabiting soil and leaf-litter environments in many parts of the world. Recent reports indicate that it is often carried by terrestrial gastropods and other small organisms in the soil habitat.

C. elegans is a small (about 1 mm long as an adult), free living (as opposed to parasitic) round worm. The normal habitat of the animal is in soil, where it feeds on bacteria and fungi. In the lab, it is grown by spreading a layer of *E. coli* onto a plate and letting the animal feed on the bacterial lawn.

Anatomy of *C. elegans* (Hermaphrodite)

C. elegans exists either as a hermaphrodite or a male. The predominant sexual form of *C. elegans* is the hermaphrodite - this animal produces both sperm and eggs. Each animal produces about 300 progeny. Self-fertilization leads to homozygosity of alleles; therefore, individual worms are considered to be genetically identical (Fig. 19).

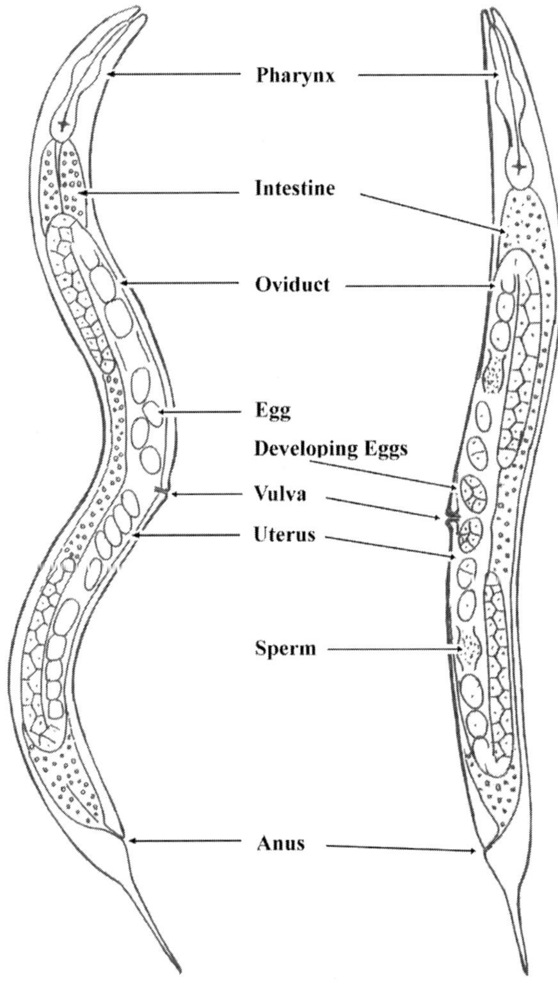

Fig. 19: Anatomy of *C. elegans* (hermaphrodite)

In *C. elegans* hermaphrodite development, there is a developmental switch- first, sperms are produced and stored in the spermatheca and then oocytes are produced. Oocyte nuclei are produced by meiotic cell division at the distal end of the gonad. They mature in a syncytium- without complete plasma membranes that separate them from one another. The nucleus and cytoplasm are completely enclosed in a plasma membrane later, just prior to fertilization. After fertilization, the eggshell is added. Fertilization takes place as maturing oocytes are squeezed through the spermatheca. Eggs develop in the hermaphrodite body briefly and then are laid through the vulva at about the 40 cell stage.

Hermaphrodites have about 10 eggs inside-the older eggs are laid about as fast as new eggs are made. Oocytes pass into the spermatheca and are fertilized. Embryos develop in the uterus and have a few cleavages before the eggs are laid, so the embryos have a few dozen cells when the embryos are laid (Fig. 20). The embryos develop into worms over the next 8-18 hours (depending on temperature).

C. elegans genotype

There are six chromosomes in *C. elegans* - five pairs of autosomes (chromosomes I, II, III, IV, V) and the sex chromosome, X (this is the letter X, not the Roman numeral ten). Hermaphrodites have two X chromosomes (designated XX). Males have one X chromosome (designated XO); having only one chromosome instead of a pair is called the hemizygous state. This state can be produced by the loss of one X chromosome or by mating. Males cannot produce progeny on their own. However, they can cross-fertilize hermaphrodites. They are commonly used in *C. elegans* genetics for making genetic combinations.

Life cycle

The life cycle is temperature-dependent. *C. elegans* goes through a reproductive life cycle (egg to egg-laying parent) in 5.5 days at 15°C, 3.5 days at 20°C and 2.5 days at 25°C.

C. elegans eggs are fertilized within the adult hermaphrodite and laid a few hours afterward- at about the 40 cell stage. Eggs hatch and animals proceed through 4 larval stages, each of which ends in a molt. When animals reach adulthood, they produce about 300 progeny each. They live for about two weeks.

C. elegans can adopt an alternative life form, called the dauer larval stage, if plates are too crowded or if food is scarce. Dauer larvae are thin and can move but their mouths are plugged and they cannot eat. Interestingly, dauers can remain viable for three months. They appear to be non-aging: dauer larvae can roam around for months and then re-enter the L4 stage when they encounter a food source and live about 15 more days.

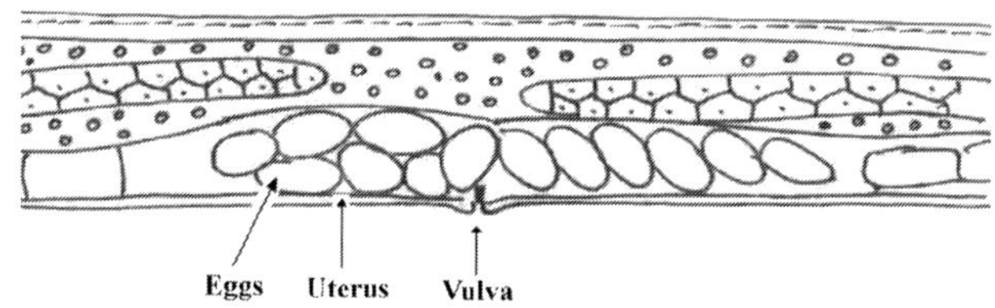

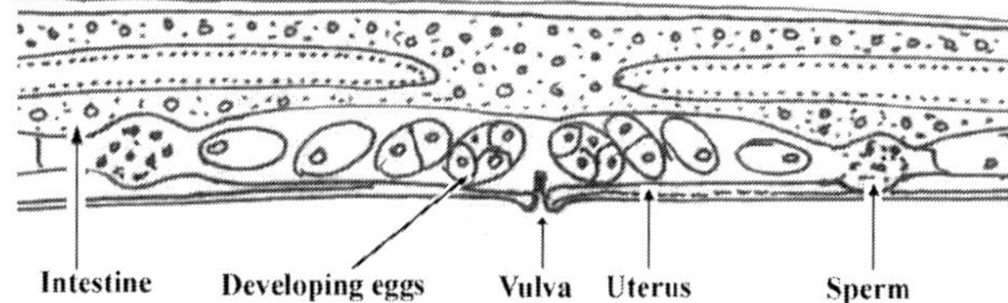

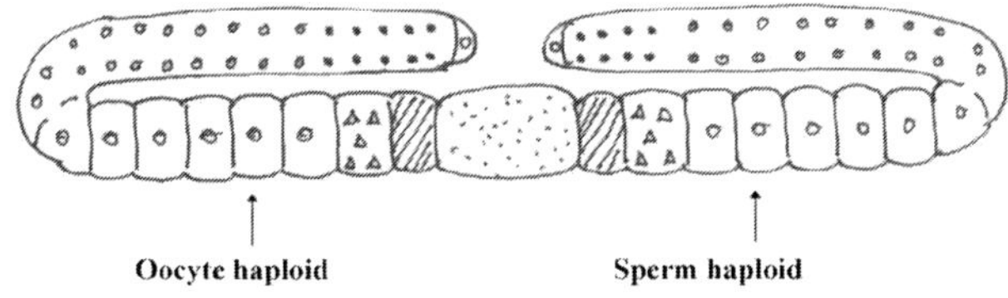

Fig. 20: Close view of hermaphrodite gonad of C. elegans

C. elegans development

C. elegans development is characterized better than any multicellular organism the complete cell lineage of the animal has been recorded. A cell lineage is a description of all the cell divisions that occur to generate a specific group of differentiated cells (in the case of *C. elegans*, the entire animal). In other words, the developmental pattern of each somatic cell is known, from the zygote to the adult worm. Thus, a scientist can identify any cell at any point in development and know the fate of that particular cell.

***C. elegans** as a biosensor*

Computer assisted video-tracking of nematodes in the presence of various toxicants using *C. elegans* as a biosensor has been developed. This assay has been used to distinguish metals, pesticides and solvents that are thought to be neurotoxins from those that are toxic but non-neuronally targeted. The researchers found significant correlation between the ranked order of toxicity on *C. elegans*, rats and mice indicating the suitability of this system for analysis of potential neurotoxicity in mammals.

While the study of xenobiotic detoxification in *C. elegans* offers a glimpse into nematode and perhaps general detoxification strategies, the system has also been tapped as a metazoan biomonitoring system. The short life cycle allows it to be utilized for rapid toxicity assessment as well as an indicator of the effects that toxicants have on subsequent generations.

Several studies have utilized reporter constructs to analyze gene expression in response to xenobiotics. Most of these studies have utilized the *LacZ reporter* gene driven by the promoter for an endogenous heat shock protein gene. One study utilized a constitutive promoter to drive expression of the bioluminescent firefly luciferase and assayed a loss of luminescence in response to temperature, metal ions and xenobiotics.

C. elegans as a biosensor offers several endpoints that can serve as markers of cellular stress, such as lethality, gene expression and behavioral changes. Assessment of lethality has been used to screen a variety of antihelmintic drugs and to test soil samples for availability of metal ions to resident nematodes. Additionally, such a system, once fully characterized, would allow the prescreening of pharmacological compounds for potential toxicity in vertebrates.

Selected References

Andersen, S. 1956. Collection of cysts of *Heterodera major* and estimation of the cyst content. *Nematologica, 1*: 303-306.

Anon, 1971. Estimated crop losses due to plant – parasitic nematodes in the United States. Special Publ. No.1, *Suppl. J. Nematol.,* 7 p.

Atkins, J.G. and Todd, E.H. 1959. White tip disease of rice, III yield tests and varietal resistance *Phytopathology, 49*: 189 – 191.

Bessey, E.A. 1911. Root – knot and its control. *U.S.D.A. Bull. 217*, 89 p.

Bhatti, D.S. and Jain, R.K. 1977. Estimation of loss in okra, tomato and brinjal yield due to *Meloidogyne incognita. Indian J. Nematol., 12* : 129 – 137.

Butler, E.J. 1913. An eelworm disease of rice. Agr. Res. Inst, Pusa, India, *Bull 34.*

Christie, J.R.1945. Some preliminary tests to determine the efficacy of certain substances when used as soil fumigants to control the root – knot nematode, *Heterodera marioni* (Cornu) Goodey. *Proc. Helminth. Soc. Wash., 12*: 14-19.

Cobb, N.A. 1914a. Nematodes and their relationships. U.S.D.A. Year Book, pp. 457 – 490.

Cobb, N.A. 1914b. The citrus – root nematode. *J. Agric. Res., 2*: 217 – 230.

Esser, R.P. and Sobers, E.K. 1964. Natural enemies of nematodes. *Proc. Soil Crop Sci. Soc. Fla., 24*: 326 – 353.

Ferris, V.R. 1971. Taxonomy of the Dorylaimida. *In: "Plant Parasitic Nematodes"* (B.M. Zuckerman,W.F. Mai and R.A. Rohde, eds.), Vol. I, pp. 164 – 189, Academic Press, New York.

Gupta, P. and Swarup, G. 1968. On the earcockle and tundu diseases of wheat. I symptoms and histopathology. *Indian Phytopath, 21:* 282 – 324.

Hewitt, W.B., Raski, D.J. and Goheen, A.C. 1958. Nematode vector of soil – borne fan leaf virus of grapevines. *Phytopathology*, *48*: 586-595.

Jones, F.G.W. 1961. The potato root eelworm, *Heterodera rostochiensis* Woll. in India *Curr. Sci., 30*: 187.

Jonathan, E.I. Gajendran, G. and Arulmozhiyan, R. 1997. Interaction of *Rotylenchulus reniformis* and *Phytophthora palmivora* in betelvine. *Nematol. Medit., 25*:9-11.

Jonathan, E.I. and Rajendran, G. 1998. Interaction of *Meloidogyne incogntia* and *Fusarium oxysporum* f.sp. *cubense* on banana. *Nematol. Medit., 26*: 9 – 11.

Jonathan, E.I. Barker, K.R. and Abd – El – Aleem, F.F. 1999. Host status of banana for four major species and host races of *Meloidogyne. Nematol. Medit., 27*: 123. 125.

Jonathan, E.I., Arulmozhiyan,R., Muthusamy, S. and Manuel. W.W. 1999. Field application of *Paecilomyces lilacinus* for the control of *Meloidogyne incognita* on betelvine. *Nematol. Medit., 28*: 131 – 133.

Jonathan,E.I., Barker, D.R., Abd – El- Aleem, F.F., Vrain,T.C. and Dickson, D.W. 2000. Biological control of *Meloidogyne incognita* on tomato and banana with rhizobacteria, Actinomycetes and *Pasteuria penetrans. Nematropica, 30*: 231-240.

Kumar, A.C., Viswanatha, P.R.K. and D'Souza, G.I. 1971. A study on plant parasitic nematodes of certain commercial crops in coffee tracts of South India. *Indian Coffee, 35*: 222-224.

Linford, M.B., and Olivera, J.M. 1938. Potential agents of biological control of plant – parasitic nematodes. *Phytopathology, 28:* 14.

Mankau, R. and Minteer, R.J.1962. Reduction of soil populations of the citrus nematode by the addition of organic materials. *Pl. Dis. Reptr., 46:* 375-378.

Nair, M.G.K., Das, N.M. and Menon, M.R. 1966. On the occurrence of the burrowing nematode, *Radopholus similis* (Cobb, 1893) Thorne, 1949 on banana in Kerala. *Indian J. Ent., 28*:553 -554.

O'Bannon, J.H. and Tomerlin, A.T. 1969. Population studies on two species of *Pratylenchus* on Citrus (Abstr.). *J. Nematol.,* 1: 299-300.

Parvatha Reddy, P. and Singh, D.B. 1978. Association of the citrus nematode with grape roots in a commercial orchard. *Curr. Sci., 47*: 640-641.

Sasser, J.N., Lucas, G.B. and Powers, H.R. 1955. The relationship of root – knot nematodes to black shank resistance in tobacco. *Phytopathology, 45*: 459 – 461.

Sivakumar, C.V. and Seshadri, A.R. 1969. Histopathology of the rice – root infested by *Hirschmanniella oryzae* (van Breda de Haan, 1902) Luc and Goodey, 1963 (Abstr.) *All India Nematol. Symp.,* New Delhi, p.1.

Thorne, G. 1961. *Principles of Nematology* McGraw-Hill, New York and London, 553 p.

Venkitesan, T.S. 1976. Studies on the burrowing nematode *Radopholus similis* (Cobb, 1893) Thorne, 1949 on pepper (*Piper nigrum* L.) and its role in slow wilt disease. *Ph.D. Thesis,* Univ. Agri. Sci., Bangalore, 122 p.

Webster, J.M. 1969. The host – parasite relationships of plant parasitic nematodes, *Advan. Parasitol., 7*:1.

Zuckerman, B.M. and Strich – Harari, D. 1964. The life stages of *Helicotylenchus multicinctus* (Cobb) in banana roots. *Nematologica, 9*: 347 – 353.

Model Questions

Chapter - II : History of Plant Nematology

I. Model Questions

1. Who is considered as the father of American Nematology?
2. The first record of plant parasitic nematode was made by _________ in the year __________.
3. Mention the contribution of the following Nematologists.

   - de Man - Carter - Atkinson

   - Christie - Goodey- Triantophyllou
4. List out the names of Nematology journals.
5. ____________ reported the potato cyst nematode for the first time from Udagamandalam, Tamil Nadu.
6. Indian Journal of Nematology was published from the year _________.
7. Centenary of Nematology in Tamil Nadu was celebrated in the year _____ at ___________ in mark of __________ .

II. Assignments

1. Name the notable nematologists in Tamil Nadu and India and mention their contributions.
2. List out the names of national and international Nematology journals.
3. Collect the name of Nematology textbooks and arrange according to their subjectwise specification.

III. For further readings

1. Dasgupta, M.K. 1996. **Phytonematology.** Nayaprakash, Calcutta, pp.846.
2. Dropkin, V.H. 1996. **Introduction to Plant Nematology** John Wiley & Sons, Newyork, pp.394.

3. Swarup, G. and Dasgupta, D.R.1986. **Plant parasitic nematodes of India : Problems and progress,** ICAR, New Delhi. pp. 521.

4. Webster, J.M. 1972. **Economic Nematology**, Academic Press, New York. pp. 238.

Chapter - III : Morphology and Anatomy of Nematodes

I. Model Questions

1. Write down the characteristics of phylum Nematoda.
2. Match the following common names of nematodes to their scientific names.

1.	Awl nematode	-	*Radopholus similis*
2.	Cyst nematode	-	*Hirschmanniella* spp.
3.	Dagger nematode	-	*Tylenchorhynchus* spp.
4.	White tip nematode	-	*Paratrichodorus* spp.,
			Trichodorus spp.
5.	Lance nematode	-	*Belonolaimus* spp.
6.	Lesion nematode	-	*Helicotylenchus* spp.
7.	Needle nematode	-	*Hemicycliophora* spp.
8.	Pin nematode	-	*Meloidogyne* spp.
9.	Reniform nematode	-	*Criconemella* spp.
10.	Ring nematode	-	*Rotylenchulus* spp.
11.	Root-knot nematode	-	*Paratylenchus* spp.
12.	Sheath nematode	-	*Longidorus* spp.
13.	Spiral nematode	-	*Pratylenchus* spp.
14.	Sting nematode	-	*Hoplolaimus* spp.
15.	Stubby-root nematodes	-	*Aphelenchoides* spp.
16.	Stunt nematode	-	*Xiphinema* spp.
17.	Rice root nematode	-	*Globodera* spp.,
			Heterodera spp.
18.	Burrowing nematode	-	*Dolichodorus* spp.

3. Describe the structure of a nematode cuticle.
4. Explain various markings on the nematode cuticle.
5. Draw a neat diagram of a typical plant parasitic nematode and label the parts.

6. Write short notes on the following

- Bursa	- Somatic musculature	- Lateral field	- Stomatostylet
- Amphid	- Striations	- Oesophagus	- Odontostylet
- Hypodermis	- Renette cell	- Phasmid	- Cardia

7. Describe the digestive system of nematodes.
8. Differentiate the male and female reproductive systems by their structure.
9. Explain the different types of nematode excretory systems.
10. Give an account on nematode sensory structures.

II. Assignments

1. Make a model of - A whole nematode
   - Typical plant parasitic nematode stylet and oesophagus
   - Sexual dimorphism
   - Feeding mechanism

III. For further readings

1. Dasgupta, M.K. 1996. **Phytonematology**. Naya Prakash, Calcutta pp.846.
2. Zuckerman, B.M., Mai, W.F. and Rohde, R.A. (Eds.) (1971). **Plant Parasitic Nematodes. Vol.I. Morphology, Anatomy, taxonomy and ecology.** Academic Press, New York and London: pp.345.

Chapter IV : Biology of Plant Parasitic Nematodes

I. Model Questions

1. Write short notes on
   - Hatching factor
   - Hatching and emergence
   - Syncytium or giant cell
   - Nurse cell
2. Describe the life cycle of any one migratory, semiendoparasitic and sedentary endoparasitic nematodes.

II. Assignments

1. Make a model of life cycle of root knot and reniform nematodes
2. Giant cell
3. Difference between root knot and bacterial nodule

III. For further readings

1. Wallace, H.R. 1963. ***Biology of Plant Parasitic Nematodes***. Arnold, London. pp. 426.

Chapter - V : Taxonomy of Plant Parasitic Nematodes

I. Model Questions

1. Give the taxonomic position of nematode.
2. Differentiate the diagnostic characters of the nematode classes Secernentea and Adenophorea.
3. Give the taxonomic position for any five important plant parasitic nematodes.

II. Assignments

1. Prepare a chart indicating taxonomical classification of economically important nematodes.
2. Differentiate the stylet and oesophagus types of Secernentea and Adenophorea.

III. For further readings

1. William, R. Nickle. 1991. **Manual of Agricultural Nematology.** Marcel Dekker Inc. New York. pp.1035.

Chapter VI : Nematological Techniques

I. Model Questions

1. What are all the different aspects to be considered while taking samples for nematode assay?
2. Describe the different methods of extraction of nematodes from soil samples with their principles.
3. How will you separate / extract nematodes from plant samples.
4. Give the procedure for staining of nematodes in plant tissue.

5. Write short notes on

   Preparation of perineal pattern
   Acid fuchsin - Lactophenol
   Numerical aperture
   Oil immersion objective

II. Assignment

1. Draw a schematic diagram for taking samples in annual and perennial crops.
2. Steps involved in microtome sectioning for histopathological studies.

III. For further readings

1. Southey, A.A.1976. Laboratory manual for soil and root nematodes. Technical Bulletin No.2. pp.74.
2. Albert, L. Taylor, 1967. **Introduction to research on Plant Nematology**. An FAO guide to the study and control of plant parasitic nematodes. Laboratory methods for nematodes. pp.174.
3. Vanfleteren, J.R. 1978. Axenic culture of free living, plant parasitic and insect parasitic nematodes. **Ann. Rev. Phytopath.** 16: 131 – 157.
4. John, E. Smith. 1996. **Biotechnology**. Cambridge University Press, Cambridge, U.K. pp.206.

Chapter - VII : Classification of Plant Parasitic Nematodes Based on their Feeding Habits

I. Model Questions

1. Explain different mode of parasitism of plant parasitic nematodes with examples.

II. Assignments

1. Foliar nematodes
2. Different types of nematode parasitism
3. Feeding by ectoparasites and others

III. For further readings

1. Nickle, W.R. 1991. **Manual of Agricultural Nematology**. Marcel Dekker inc. New york. pp.940.

Chapter - VIII : Nematode Disease Symptoms on Crop Plants

I. Model Questions

1. Write short notes on the following symptoms of damage.

- Blind plant	- Dieback	- Red ring of coconut
- Day wilting	- Lesions	- Root gall
- Stubby root	- Fishhook	- Stunting and Patchiness

II. Assignments

1. Prepare a chart mentioning different nematode disease of crops and nematodes responsible for the same and indicate yield loss nationally and globally.

III. For further readings

1. Siddique, M.R. 1993. **Tylenchida parasites of plants and animals.** CAB. International Academic Press pp.340.

Chapter - IX : Interaction of Nematodes with Microorganisms

I. Model Questions

1. What is meant by nematode disease complex? Mention the role of associated organisms.
2. Give examples for economically important
   a. Nematode fungal disease complex
   b. Nematode bacterial disease complex
   c. Nematode viral disease complex in Tamil Nadu, India and worldwide

II. Assignments

1. Describe the mechanism of virus transmission by nematodes.
2. Physiological, histopathological and biochemical changes induced by nematode alone and nematode disease complex

III. For further readings

1. Powell, N.T. 1971. **Interaction of plant parasitic nematodes with other disease causing agents.** Plant Parasitic nematodes Vol.II Eds.B.M. Zuckerman, W.F. Mai and R.A. Rohde. Academic press. pp.347.
2. Wajid Khan, M. 1993. **Nematode Interactions** Chapman & Hall. pp.377.

3. Brown, D.J.F., Robertson, W.M. and Trudgill, D.L. 1995. Transmission of viruses by plant nematodes. **Ann. Rev. Phytopath**. 33:223 -250.

4. Powell, N.T. 1971. Interactions between nematodes and fungi in disease complex. **Ann. Rev. Phytopath.** (9) 253-274.

5. Mai, W.F. and Abawi. G.S. 1987. Interactions among root-knot nematodes and Fusarium wilt fungi on host plants. **'Ann. Rev. Phytopath.** 25: 317.

Chapter - X : Nematode Pests of Field Crops

I. Model Questions

1. List out the nematodes associated with rice with their symptoms of damage and their management practices.

2. Write short notes on

    i. White tip disease of rice

    ii. Molya disease

    iii. Ear cockle

    iv. Tundu disease

3. Mention about symptomology, biology, ecology of *Anguina tritici* and how will you manage the nematode by Integrated nematode management practices.

II. Assignments

i. Physical and

ii. Cultural methods suggested for the management of rice and wheat nematodes.

III. For further readings

1. Bhatti, D.S. and Walia, R.K. 1989. **Nematode pests of crops** pp. 423.

2. Luc, M., Sikora, R.A. and Bridge. J. 1990. **Plant parasitic nematodes in subtropical and tropical agriculture.** CAB International Institute of Parasitology, UK pp.629.

3. Trivedi, P.C. 1998. **Nematode Diseases in Plants**. CBS Publishers and Distributors, New Delhi, pp. 414.

4. Evans, K., Trudgill, D.L. and Webster. Jon. 1996. **Plant parasitic nematodes in Temperate Agriculture,** CAB International, Wallingford, UK pp. 647.

Chapter - XI : Nematode Pests of Fruit Crops

I. Model Questions

1. Mention the name of the nematodes responsible for the following disease and how will you diagnose the diseases.
   i. Slow decline
   ii. Toppling disease
2. Write an essay on nematodes of grapevine and papaya, their symptoms of damage and management practices.
3. Nematodes are serious biotic stress in banana - Discuss.

II. Assignment

1. How will you diagnose the different nematode damage in citrus, banana, grapevine and papaya?

III. For further readings

1. Luc, M., Richard A. Sikora and Bridge 1990. J. **Plant parasitic nematodes in sub tropical and tropical agriculture**. CAB International Institute of Parasitology UK pp.629.

Chapter - XII : Nematode Pests of Vegetable Crops

I. Model Questions

1. Write short notes on
   i. White females
   ii. Nematode wool
2. Write down the symptomology, ecology and biology of PCN and suggest suitable remedial measure to contain the nematode problem.
3. List out nematodes associated with important vegetable crops.
4. How will you manage nematode problems by different methods of nematode management practices in vegetable crops.

II. Assignment

1. Recommended package of practices for the management of potato and vegetable nematodes with special reference to biological control.

III. For further readings

1. Luc, M., Richard A. Sikora and Bridge. J. 1990. **Plant parasitic nematodes in sub tropical and tropical Agriculture**. CAB international Institute of Parasitology UK pp.629.
2. Gopal Swarup, Dasgupta, D.R. and Gill, J.S. 1995. **Nematode Pest Management** : An Appraisal of Ecofriendly Approaches. Nematological Society of India, New Delhi, pp. 300.

Chapter - XIII : Nematode Pests of Commercial Flower Crops

I. Model Questions

1. Mention different nematodes associated with crossandra, tuberose and jasmine.
2. Brief about nematode fungal disease complex in crossandra and jasmine.
3. How will you manage nematode and nematode disease complex in crossandra, tuberose and jasmine?

II. Assignments

1. Draw symptoms of nematode damage in flower crops grown commonly in your areas.

III. For further readings

1. Luc, M., Richard A. Sikora and Bridge. J. 1990. **Plant parasitic nematodes in sub tropical and tropical Agriculture**. CAB international Institute of Parasitology UK pp.629.

Chapter - XIV . Nematode Pests of Spices and Plantation Crops

I. Model Questions

1. Mention the key nematode pests of the following crops in Tamil Nadu.

Blackpepper	Cardamom	Turmeric	Arecanut
Coffee	Tea	Betelvine	

2. How will you manage tea nematodes in nursery and main field?
3. Mention about geographical distribution, symptoms, life cycle, host range of *Pratylenchus coffeae* and management practices in coffee.
4. Suggest integrated nematode management practices for the management of nematodes in turmeric.

II. Assignments

1. Tabulate the associated nematodes, symptoms of damage and management practices in spices and plantation crops.

III. For further readings

1. Luc, M., Richard, A. Sikora and Bridge, J. 1990. **Plant parasitic nematodes in sub tropical and tropical agriculture.** CAB International Institute of Parasitology UK pp.629.

Chapter - XV : Nematode Pests of Medicinal and Aromatic Plants

I. Model Questions

1. Mention about nematodes associated with Dioscorea, their symptoms of damage and measures suggested to overcome the nematode infestation.

II. Assignments

1. Quantitative and qualitative economic yield loss due to nematodes in medicinal and aromatic plants.

III. For further readings

1. Evans, K., Trudgill, D.L. and Webster. J.M. 1991. **Plant parasitic nematodes in temperate agriculture**. CAB international, Walling ford, UK pp.647.

Chapter - XVI : Nematode Control

I. Model Questions

1. Why regulatory control is considered as a first line of defense in nematode management? Support with suitable examples.
2. Mention about domestic and foreign quarantine acts with suitable examples.
3. Write short notes on
   i. DIP
   ii. Prevention of nematode spread / multiplication
4. Give suitable examples for the physical method of nematode management.
5. What is the principle of the following cultural methods of nematode management?

   i. Selection of healthy seed material
   ii. Adjusting the time of planting
   iii. Fallowing and summer ploughing
   iv. Flooding
   v. Trap / antagonistic crops

6. Critically discuss about the feasibility of biological control of nematodes.
7. Mention about the available chemical nematicides and their methods of treatment and application.

II. Assignment

1. Bioagents and their commercial formulations recommended against plant parasitic nematodes.

III. For further readings

1. Bridge, J. Nematode management in sustainable and subsistence agriculture. Ann. Rev. Phytopath. 34: 201-226.
2. Larry W. Duncan. 1991. 'Current options for nematode management'. Ann. Rev. Phytopath.29. pp.469.
3. Sikora, R.A. 1992. Management of the antagonistic potential in agricultural ecosystems for the biological control of plant-parasitic nematodes. Ann. Rev. Phytopath. 30:245-270.
4. Jatala, P. 1986. Biological control of plant parasitic nematodes. Ann. Rev Phytopath.24:453-489.
5. Singh, S.B. and S. Hussain. 1998. Biological suppression of plant diseases, phytoparasitic nematodes and weeds, Project Directorate of Biological Control, Bangalore. pp.79.
6. Brown, R.H. and Kerry, B.R. 1993. Principles and practices of nematode control in crops. Academic Press, New York. pp. 437.
7. Gopal Swarup, Dasgupta, D.R. and Gill, J.S. 1995. Nematode Pest Management : An Appraisal of Ecofriendly Approaches. Nematological Society of India, New Delhi, pp. 300.

Colour Plates

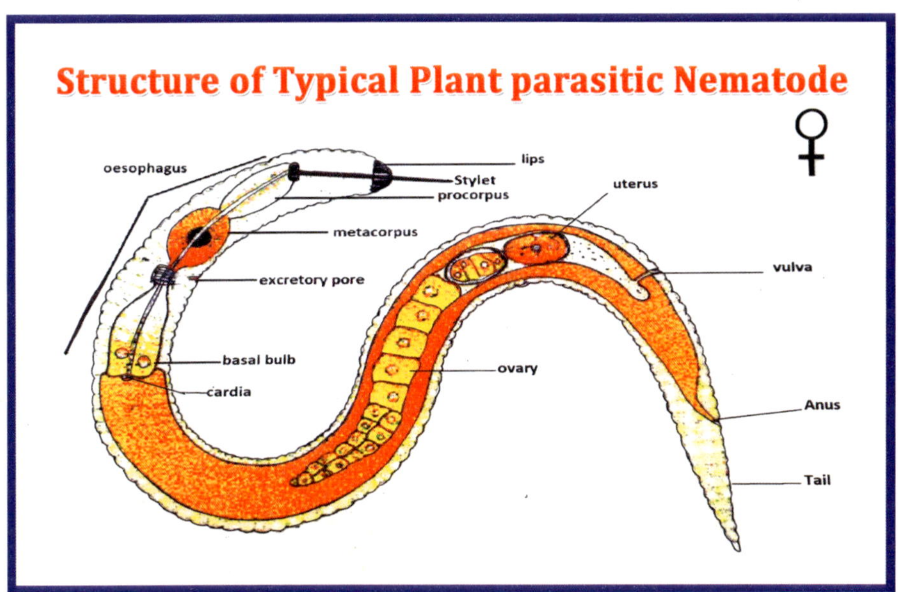

Fig. 1: Morphology of a typical plant parasitic nematode

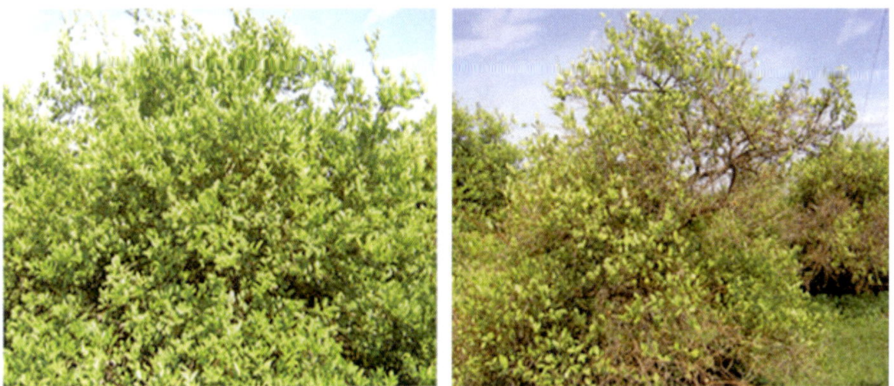

Plate 3: Citrus tree infested with T. semipenetrans

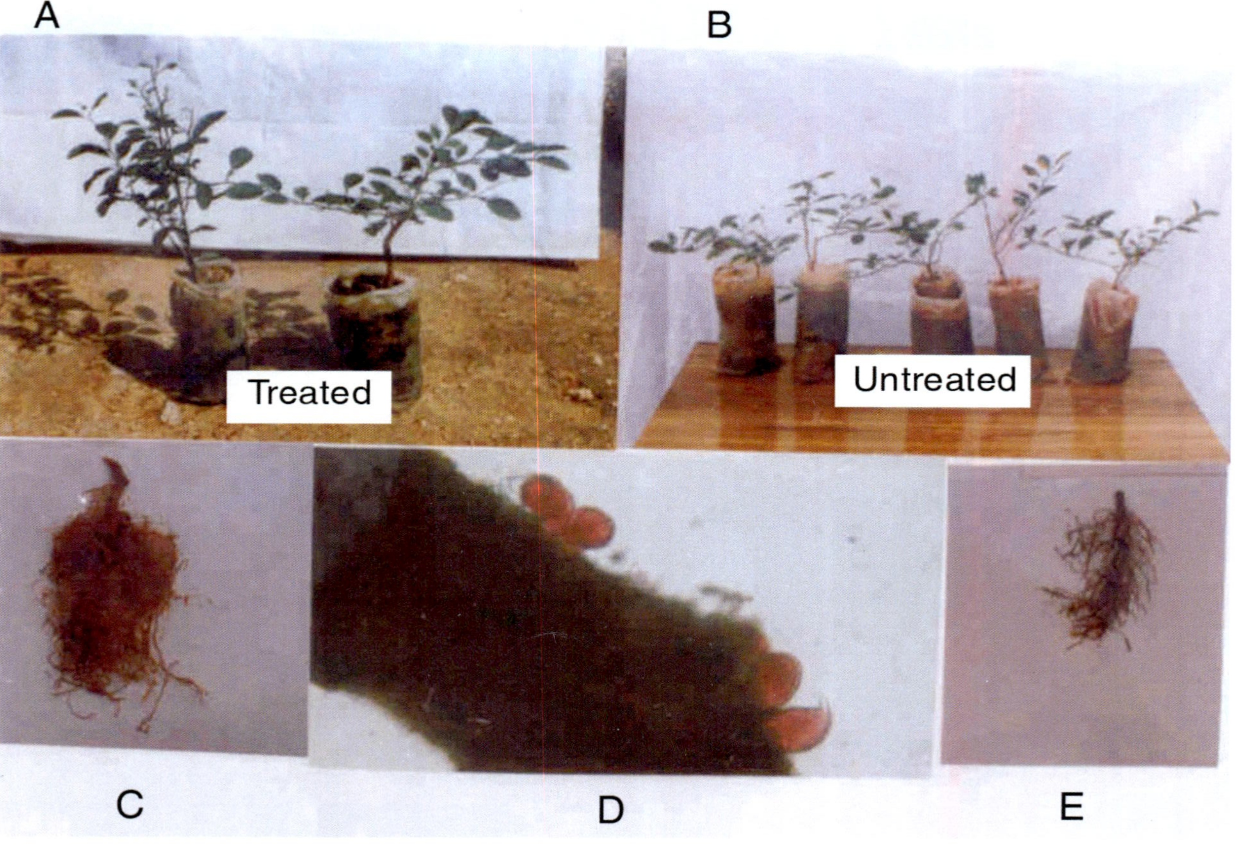

Plate 4: A. Healthy seedling **B**. Infested seedling **C**. Healthy seedling root **D**. Affected root **E**. Females attached to citrus root

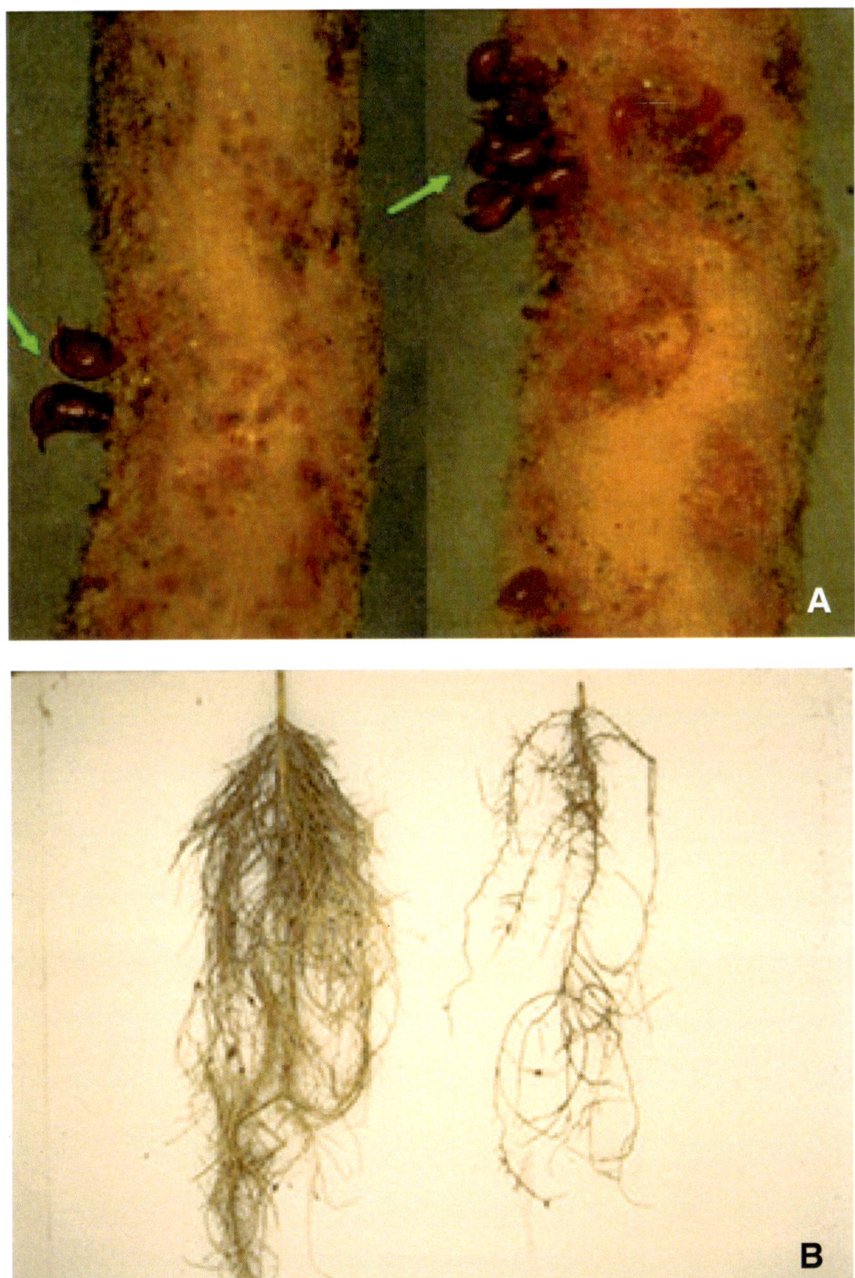

Plate 4: A. Females attached to roots **B.** Healthy and infested seedling roots

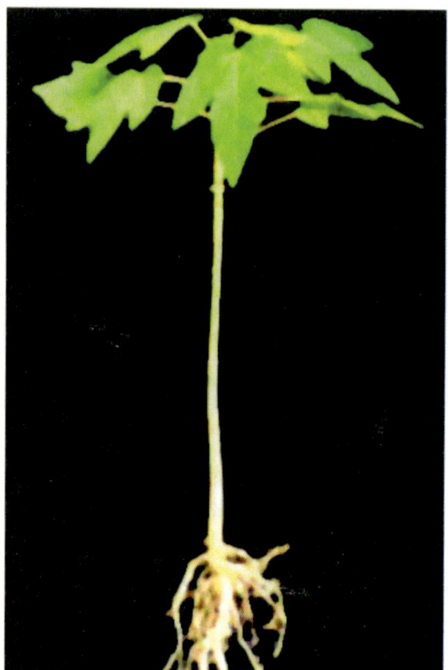

Plate 6: Papaya seedling infested with root-knot nematode

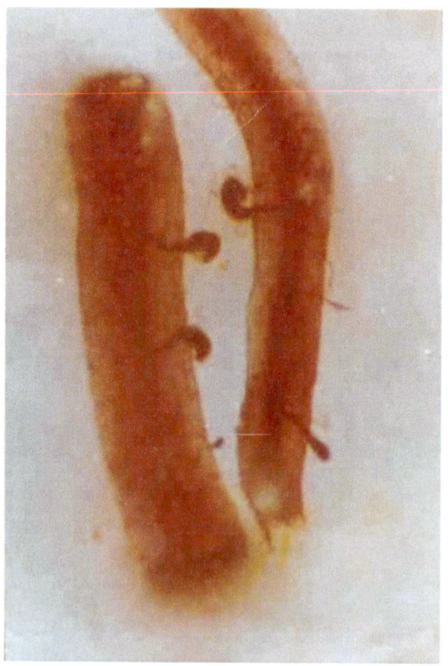

Plate 7: Papaya root infested with reniform nematode (reniform females attached to the root as semiendoparasite)